618.97

Guidelines on Depression in Older People

Practising the Evidence

KT-569-755

Prepared under the auspices of the World Psychiatric Association Sections of Old Age Psychiatry and Affective Disorders

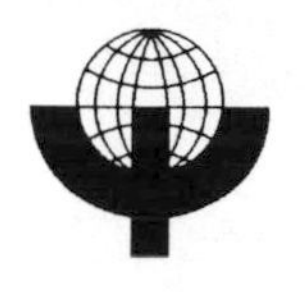

LIBRARY & INFORMATION SERVICE
TEES, ESK & WEAR VALLEYS
NHS FOUNDATION TRUST
CROSS LANE HOSPITAL
SCARBOROUGH

Guidelines on Depression in Older People

Practising the Evidence

Robert C Baldwin DM FRCP FRCPsych
Consultant Psychiatrist and Honorary Professor of Old Age Psychiatry
University of Manchester
Manchester Mental Health and Social Care Trust
Manchester Royal Infirmary
Manchester
UK

Edmond Chiu AM MBBS DPM FRANZCP
Associate Professor in Psychiatry of Old Age
Academic Unit for Psychiatry of Old Age
University of Melbourne
St George's Health Service
Kew, Victoria
Australia

Cornelius Katona MD FRCPsych
Professor of Psychiatry of the Elderly
University College London
London
UK

Nori Graham Bm BCh FRCPsych DUniv
Emeritus Consultant in Old Age Psychiatry
Royal Free Hospital
London
UK

informa
HEALTHCARE

© 2002, 2006 Informa Healthcare, an imprint of Informa UK Limited

First published in the United Kingdom in 2002 by Martin Dunitz Ltd.

This edition published by Informa Healthcare, an imprint of Informa UK Limited,
2 Park Square, Milton Park, Abingdon, Oxon OX14 4RN

Tel: +44 (0)20 7017 6000
Fax: +44 (0)20 7017 6699
Email: info.medicine@tandf.co.uk
Website: www.tandf.co.uk/medicine

All rights reserved. No part of this publication may be reproduced, stored in a retrieval system, or transmitted, in any form or by any means, electronic, mechanical, photocopying, recording, or otherwise, without the prior permission of the publisher or in accordance with the provisions of the Copyright, Designs and Patents Act 1988 or under the terms of any licence permitting limited copying issued by the Copyright Licensing Agency, 90 Tottenham Court Road, London W1P 0LP.

Although every effort has been made to ensure that all owners of copyright material have been acknowledged in this publication, we would be glad to acknowledge in subsequent reprints or editions any omissions brought to our attention.

A CIP record for this book is available from the British Library.
Library of Congress Cataloging-in-Publication Data

Data available on application

ISBN-10: 1 84184 126 9
ISBN-13: 978 1 84184 126 7

Distributed in North and South America by
Taylor & Francis
6000 Broken Sound Parkway, NW, (Suite 300)
Boca Raton, FL 33487, USA

Within Continental USA
Tel: 1 (800) 272 7737; Fax: 1 (800) 374 3401
Outside Continental USA
Tel: (561) 994 0555; Fax: (561) 361 6018
Email: orders@crcpress.com

Distributed in the rest of the world by
Thomson Publishing Services
Cheriton House
North Way
Andover, Hampshire SP10 5BE, UK
Tel: +44 (0)1264 332424
Email: tps.tandfsalesorder@thomson.com

Composition by Wearset Ltd, Boldon, Tyne and Wear
Printed and bound by Antony Rowe Ltd, Eastbourne

Contents

Introduction

Worldwide, life expectancy is increasing. Currently about 10% of the world's population is made up of older adults (aged 65 and above). This figure is set to rise steadily, to as much as 30% in some societies (Moussaoui, 1999). For mental health this will mean an increase not only in the neurodegenerative conditions, such as Alzheimer's disease, but also of depressive disorder. This affects about one in 10 people aged over 65, making it the most common of the mental health disorders of later life.

In recognition of the global impact of depressive disorder, the World Psychiatric Association (WPA) commissioned a major initiative under the banner title of Prevention and Treatment of Depression (PTD), bringing together psychiatrists from around the world. The teaching modules that arose from the PTD venture, one of which specifically addresses later life, are available on the WPA website: http://www.wpanet.org/sectorial/edu4.html. In another WPA initiative a major review of the evidence concerning all facets of depressive disorder was undertaken. This has been published in book form under the title *Depressive Disorders*, and includes a major review of depressive disorder in later life (Chiu et al, 1999). The International Psychogeriatric Association (IPA) too has acknowledged the importance of depressive disorder by establishing a Mood Disorders Task Force.

The message from these initiatives is clear: there is robust evidence showing that depressive disorder in later life is treatable, and that the benefits of treatment, for the individual, families and society, are immense. Yet research continues to highlight low levels of detection and treatment, especially in primary care. It seems that there is a gap between knowing the evidence and implementing it. This book presents a further development in WPA's strategy and has been prepared under the auspices of the WPA sections for Old Age Psychiatry and Affective Disorders. The aim is to bridge the gap between knowledge and practice by providing a concise summary of available evidence which will then serve as guidance for practice.

Cole and Yaffe (1996), modifying an adaptation of a pathways model, estimated that only about one in 10 older people with depression in the community are referred for psychiatric care. Therefore the focus of this book is primary care, because that is the setting where most depressive disorder occurs and is managed. However, we have included sufficient detail so that it will be of interest to psychiatrists, neurologists and specialists in geriatric medicine (including those in training), as well as nurses and other practitioners whose work involves older people and who wish to update their knowledge from a sound evidence base. The busy reader can refer to the summary boxes and recommendations and those who wish for more detail will find it in the text.

It would be impossible in a short book to document all the evidence that exists on the topic of late-life depression; nor is there any need to, as there are excellent reviews and articles. Our approach therefore has been to start with key documents in which we believe the most important evidence has already been summarised. Two of these have already been referred to: the WPA Prevention and Treatment of Depression (PTD) Module for the Elderly, published in 1999, and the review published as a book chapter in *Depressive Disorders*, commissioned by the World Psychiatric Association. Also included are the British Association of Psychopharmacology (BAP) updated evidence-based guidelines (Anderson et al, 2000); the National Institutes of Health Diagnosis and Treatment of Depression in Later Life Consensus Statement, published in book form in 1991, summarised in the *Journal of the American Medical Association* in 1992 and updated in 1997; and lastly, *Pharmacotherapy of Depressive Disorders in Older Patients*, the findings of an expert group from the United States (Alexopoulos et al, 2001). These references are listed in Appendix A, and are referred to in the text by abbreviations: PTD, WPA, BAP, NIH and EXP, respectively.

One of the authors, RCB, then conducted a literature search on MEDLINE, EMBASE, Cinahl and Psychinfo databases for the years 1998–October 2001 inclusive. This period was chosen because two of the key documents, NIH and WPA, were current to the years 1997 and 1998, respectively. The search strategy used all the terms relevant to depressive disorder and dysthymia combined with the keywords 'aged', 'elderly', 'geriatric' and 'senile'. The reliability of the search was examined by cross-checking all 1998 references from the WPA document with the new search to see if it had detected them; it had. Only original research papers were included in the search. The 1000 or so articles were then organised under the chapter headings matching those of the PTD initiative. A list of evidence-based statements, i.e. those supported by the existing literature and the new search, was then drawn up by RCB and circulated for comment to the other authors. This cycle was repeated, with the agreed levels of evidence and recommendations for practice (see below) added on the last cycle.

In order to prioritise the evidence we have used a widely adopted grading of evidence, along with recommendations that follow from this (after Shekelle et al, 1999, and adopted by Anderson et al, 2000, BAP). This is summarised in Box 0.1. Levels of evidence are specified, with the highest level accorded to meta-analyses of randomised controlled trials. An alphabetical grading system, A–D, is then applied to arrive at the overall strength of recommendations. However, the latter reflects the evidence on which it is based, not necessarily its importance in practice. Recommendations with a weaker evidence base are often helpful in addressing areas where clinical decisions have to be made. We are also conscious that this system lends itself less well to some areas of research such as epidemiological and cohort studies and that there is therefore a tendency to artificially down-rate evidence of this kind.

The structure of each chapter begins with factual information about the evidence, then a summary box of evidence-based statements, followed by recommendations for practice. At the end of each chapter we highlight newer, emerging themes and questions for the future. We

Box 0.1 Categories of evidence and strength of recommendations

Categories of evidence for causal relationships and treatment
(Shekelle et al, 1999)

- Ia Evidence from meta-analysis of randomised controlled trials
- Ib Evidence from at least one randomised controlled trial
- IIa Evidence from at least one controlled study without randomisation
- IIb Evidence from at least one other type of quasi-experimental study
- III Evidence from non-experimental descriptive studies, such comparative studies, correlation studies and case–control studies
- IV Evidence from expert committees reports or opinions and/or clinical experience of respected authorities

Strength of recommendation

- A Directly based on category I evidence
- B Directly based on category II evidence or extrapolated recommendation from category I evidence
- C Directly based on category III evidence or extrapolated recommendation from category I or II evidence
- D Directly based on category IV evidence or extrapolated recommendation from category I, II or III evidence.

hope that this approach will also serve to highlight research priority areas.

Clearly it is not possible to cite all the references that were scrutinised, but we have listed some of the more important and/or illustrative ones, along with others that seem to represent potentially important avenues for future inquiry. These are listed alphabetically in Appendix B. Most of the references in this list are newer, but some older work is cited as needed, although we have kept referencing of this kind to a minimum as there are a number of good general texts (listed in Appendix C) that discuss classic or older material. For busy clinicians, and as a quick reference, we have reproduced the evidence boxes and recommendations in the Executive summary.

We are aware that books written by experts sometimes contain more dogma and opinion than fact. Throughout we have tried to avoid making statements that cannot be backed by evidence. Where there are issues which are uncertain or which remain unresolved, we have tried to make that clear.

chapter 1

Signs and symptoms of depression in later life

The symptoms of depressive disorder

In Box 1.1, taken from ICD10 (WHO, 1993), the features of depressive disorder are listed under core symptoms and additional symptoms. Similar symptoms are used in DSMIV (American Psychiatric Association). The following distinguish major depressive disorder from understandable sadness:

- *Duration:* symptoms are present for at least 2 weeks;
- *Lack of fluctuation:* symptoms occur on most days, most of the time;
- *Intensity:* must be of a degree that is definitely not normal for that individual.

In addition to these, in classifactory systems such as ICD10 and DSMIV whether or not an individual can be said to have depressive disorder is determined by (a) the presence and number of *core* symptoms, and (b) the number of *additional* symptoms.

- For *mild* depressive episode:
  - Two core symptoms
  - At least four additional symptoms
- For *moderate* depressive episode:
  - Two core symptoms
  - At least six additional symptoms

Box 1.1 Main features of depressive disorder

Core symptoms

- Depressed mood sustained for at least 2 weeks
- Loss of interest or pleasure in normal activities
- Decreased energy, increased fatigue

Additional symptoms

- Loss of confidence or self-esteem
- Inappropriate and excessive guilt
- Recurrent thoughts of death; suicidal thoughts or behaviour
- Diminished evidence of ability to think or concentrate, e.g. indecisiveness
- Change in psychomotor activity
- Sleep disturbance
- Appetite change with corresponding weight change

WPA Prevention & Treatment of Depression Module 3 (PTD)

- For *severe* depressive episode:
  - All three core symptoms
  - At least five additional symptoms
  - A further subdivision may be made depending on the presence or absence of psychotic symptoms and/or stupor.

In addition to symptoms of depression the individual will also have some degree of incapacity as a result of being depressed. This will vary in intensity, but will be marked in the severest forms of depression (BAP).

The clinical picture in late-life depressive disorder

Major depression in older people is essentially the same disorder as at other times of life. It is untrue that depressive disorder in an older person cannot be distinguished from normal ageing (NIH). There is insufficient evidence to suggest that there is a subtype of major depression unique to older people, although there is rather more evidence in favour of a subtype of non-major depression – so-called minor depression, which will be discussed in Chapter 3. Rather, ageing may accentuate some clinical features of depressive disorder and suppress others. Current evidence points to the following as factors that may modify the clinical manifestation of later-life depressive disorder:

- When depressed, today's older people complain less often of sadness than their younger contemporaries, and this does not appear to be simply a cohort effect (NIH).
- Hypochondriasis is consistently reported as a symptom more common in later-life depression (NIH).
- Subjective memory complaint may be a leading symptom of depression in the aged. The literature points to a strong correlation between depressed mood and subjective memory complaint, especially in the 'younger' elderly (65–75 years). In patients referred to memory clinics about a fifth of those who present with a memory complaint will, upon investigation, be found to have a depressive disorder rather than a dementia.
- Anxiety is a common accompaniment of depression in later life. When it dominates the clinical picture an underlying depression may be overlooked (see also Chapter 6, Comorbidity).
- There is emerging evidence that patients with brain injury from a variety of causes may display apathy as a prominent symptom, and that although there is overlap between apathy and depression, the two can be distinguished clinically (Andersson et al, 1999). For example, patients with apathy have low motivation as a symptom rather than anhedonia, and have fewer depressive thoughts (NIH). Apathy is more likely to respond to behavioural than to antidepressant intervention.
- Dementia may alter the presentation of depression. For example, behavioural symptoms such as disruptive vocalisation have been found to be more prominent than depressive thoughts such as guilt and worthlessness (Dwyer & Byrne, 2000).
- Impaired cognition is not uncommon in depression. In moderately ill patients it may cause impairment in complex tasks and timed tests (Palsson et al, 2000), and in severe depression it may produce a

picture similar to a dementia (sometimes referred to a 'pseudodementia'). It is possible that the hippocampus, the seat of memory, becomes damaged in some patients with chronic depression, perhaps as a result of persistently elevated endogenous steroid levels (Steffens et al, 2000; Ashatri et al, 1999).

Summary of evidence

- In older people depressive disorder can be distinguished from normal ageing (IIa)
- Major depressive disorder in older people often manifests in the same way as in younger adults (IIa)
- There is little evidence of a specific subtype of major depression in older people (IIa)
- But several factors modify its presentation (IIb). These include:
  - A reduced complaint of sadness
  - Hypochondriasis and somatic concern instead of sadness
  - Poor subjective memory or a dementia-like picture
  - Marked anxiety
  - Apathy and poor motivation

Recommendations for practice

- In order to detect major depression in older people, it is important that practitioners are trained to recognise the leading symptoms as outlined in major classificatory systems such as ICD10 and DSM IV (B)
- Equally it is important to be aware of symptoms which are often the clue to an underlying depression in an older person. The most important of these are:
  - a reduced complaint of sadness, even when appearing depressed to others
  - excessive preoccupation with health and physical symptoms
  - when the patient is distressed by poor memory rather than depression (B)

Newer themes and issues for future research

Cultural factors may also modify the presentation of depressive disorder. For example, it has been said that older depressed people from Southeast Asia often present with a physical complaint without depressed mood. However, in one recent epidemiological study that used a widely known screening instrument, the CES-D, to assess depression, there appeared to be a core of depressive symptoms which were common to several different Asian cultures and which were similar to those found in North America (Mackinnon et al, 1998). Cultural modification of depressive disorder is an important topic of ongoing research.

chapter 2

Disease burden

Depressive disorder is a global health problem. According to the World Health Organization (1999) by 2020 depression will be the leading illness associated with negative impact and disease burden. This is true of all adult age groups but the following facts, several derived from recent evidence, are pertinent to depressive disorder in later life:

- As a cause of morbidity depression already ranks alongside the eight most disabling medical conditions, including heart disease (NIH).
- It leads to inappropriate use of hospital beds (Ingold et al, 2000); and
- It leads to a greater risk of hospitalisation (Huang et al, 2000).
- It is the single most important predictor of suicide in older people (NIH, WPA, PTD).
- It is a cause of disability in its own right; it also adds to disability from physical disorder when present and leads to greater physical decline (Penninx et al, 2000).
- It prolongs periods of hospitalisation for physical disorder (NIH).
- It leads to reduced compliance with medical treatments (NIH).
- It reduces quality of life (NIH, PTD).
- It is an independent predictor of mortality (NIH, PTD).
- It increases healthcare utilisation costs (NIH).
- Patients with bipolar disorder (although this is relatively uncommon in later life), consume approximately four times more mental health care than those with unipolar depression (Bartels et al, 2000).

Depressive disorder in older people is underdiagnosed in primary care, hospital medical facilities for older people and nursing and residential care homes (NIH, PTD). Furthermore, there is evidence from epidemiological studies (NIH, WPA, PTD) that the use of antidepressants among older depressed people in the community is as low as one in 10; that for tricyclic antidepressants about half the prescriptions are subtherapeutic; and that the use of (generally inappropriate) benzodiazepines is comparatively high.

It is important not to allow such bleak facts to overwhelm the practitioner, for recent evidence also shows that when older patients with depression are treated they enjoy an unequivocally improved quality of life (Shmuely et al, 2001). Yet it is likely that one reason why depressive disorder continues to cause such a huge public health burden despite an overall improvement in general health care in many countries is because its true impact is consistently ignored or underestimated.

Summary of evidence

- As a cause of suffering, depressive disorder is one of the leading causes worldwide (IIa)
- It is often not recognised or is inadequately treated (IIa)
- As a result it increases morbidity from associated conditions, pushes up costs and hastens death (IIa)
- With appropriate treatment, quality of life for the older person is improved (Ib)

Recommendations for practice

- The enormous negative impact of depressive disorder in older people should be acknowledged in government policy and health planning (B)
- Practitioners should regard depressive disorder in older people as a serious and potentially chronic condition, like other seriously disabling conditions (B)
- Practitioners should have a low threshold for its detection, as it is frequently overlooked (B)
- Practitioners should become familiar with its management, as it is often not treated optimally (B)

Newer themes and issues for future research

- There is emerging evidence that some patients with major depression in later life have brain dysfunction which results in a dysexecutive syndrome (a form of frontal lobe disorder causing problems with mental flexibility), and that this may be an important additional cause of disability (Kiosses et al, 2000).
- Patients with severe depression, such as those admitted to psychiatric care, usually meet criteria for major depressive episode (as in ICD10). However, population studies reveal a different picture. For example, in one such study an alternative criterion-based system for depression in older people was developed which deliberately excluded dysphoria as one of its symptoms. Those patients who were 'non-dysphorically' depressed suffered significant distress, disability and a higher mortality despite not meeting criteria for major depression (Stage et al, 2001). Data from large epidemiological studies have become available in recent years. The direction this seems to be pointing in is that in order to understand the burden of depression it is important to study the full range of depressive disorders and not, as was previously the case, restrict enquiry only to major depression.

chapter 3

Types of depressive disorder in later life

If a patient has at least five symptoms (including two core ones) from the list in Box 1.1, then by definition he or she has a 'major' depressive episode. On the whole, the evidence suggests that the ICD10 and DSMIV concept of major depression is applicable to older people in that both younger and older people diagnosed with major depression have very similar symptomatologies (Stage et al, 2001). However, this may be tautological, as the use of rigid diagnostic criteria risks defining away those features that may be specific for older adults. This accords with the epidemiological evidence, which shows that typical major depression accounts for only between one-quarter and a third of older people with significant depressive symptomatology (see Chapter 4 (NIH, WPA)).

There is no consensus as to what to call depression that is non-major, although terms such as 'subthreshold' depression, 'subclinical' depression, 'minor' depression, dysthymia and 'milder' depression have all been used.

Recent evidence suggests that:

- 'Minor' and 'major' depression in older people share similar risk factors, such as poor health, isolation, disablement and poor satisfaction with life (WPA, NIH);
- Both 'minor' and 'major' depressive disorder are similarly associated with
  - reduced physical activity

  - less social contact, and
  - higher mortality (NIH, WPA, PTD);
- Subsyndromal/minor depressive disorder/non-major depression is associated with functional impairment of a similar magnitude to major depression (Lyness et al, 1999b);
- In mixed-aged samples, having non-major depression is a risk factor for 'major' depression (NIH);
- In mixed-aged samples, a sizeable proportion of non-major depression is due to incomplete resolution of symptoms in patients with major depression (NIH).

One study spanning several European countries used a statistical technique to group a broad range of depressive symptoms identified in community-dwelling older people. Unlike ICD and DSM it did not make *a priori* assumptions about them. Two groups of symptoms were identified:

- 'Affective suffering', characterised by depression, tearfulness and a wish to die; and
- A 'motivation' factor, comprising loss of interest, poor concentration and anhedonia.

Box 3.1 Classification of depressive disorder

Major depression

- Depressive episode (mild, moderate, severe) (ICD F32.0,1.2)
- Major depressive disorder (DSM 296)
- Recurrent depressive disorder (ICD F33.0,1,2)

Non-major (subthreshold) depression

- Minor depression (DSM IV)
- Dysthymia (DSM IV 300.4, ICD F34.1)
- Adjustment disorder with depressed mood (DSM 309, ICD F43.2)
- Mixed anxiety and depressive disorder (ICD F41.2, DSM IV)
- Milder depression (BAP)

In another study, Blazer (1991) identified a cluster of depressive symptoms unique to community-dwelling people aged over 60 characterised by:

- Low mood
- Psychomotor retardation
- Poor concentration
- Constipation
- Poor perceived health
- Cognitive deficits
- An association with physical ill-health.

These lines of evidence strengthen the view that current classificatory systems such as ICD10 and DSMIV, with their emphasis on minimum symptom counts to denote a 'case', overlook clinically significant depressive states in older people. Furthermore, these data suggest there may be a distinct form of depressive disorder in later life characterised less by low mood and depressive ideation than by low motivation, poor concentration, retardation and physical ill-health.

The term minor depression has recently become popular and is used in two main ways: (i) to denote depressive states with substantially the same sort of symptoms as major depression but fewer of them; and (ii) to characterise a syndrome with different symptoms from major depression. What has become clear is that 'minor' depression is not a trivial or unimportant mood state. For a review of minor depression in older people see Tannock and Katona (1995). In this book we use the term minor depression interchangeably with subthreshold depression, non-major depression and subclinical depression. The prevalence of minor depression increases with age in an approximately linear fashion, and it therefore becomes the most common depressive disorder of older people (NIH).

For simplicity we have divided depressive states into two groups, major and non-major depression (Box 3.1). Some features of minor depression are listed in Box 3.2. However, it is clear that the nosology of depressive disorder in later life requires further clarification.

Box 3.2 'Minor' depression

- Is the most common depressive disorder of older people
- Is associated with the same negative effects as major depression
- Is certainly not trivial
- Is commonly associated with physical ill-health
- And may have a characteristic symptom profile with amotivation, poor concentration and poorer cognition

Other types of depressive disorder that affect older people

- If a depression is due to the effects of a systemic disorder and/or drug, the term *organic mood (depressive) disorder* is used. The criteria for major depression still have to be met. The causes of organic mood disorder are discussed in Chapter 5. Organic mood disorder is more frequent in older than in younger depressed patients (PTD).
- Depression may occur as part of *bipolar disorder*, although the usual onset for this is in younger adulthood. Onset in later life is often associated with organic brain disease and considerable morbidity.
- *Dysthymia* is a chronic disorder of mood characterised by several symptoms of depression, usually insufficient to meet 'case' level as in ICD or DSM depressive episode or major depression, with some fluctuation. Duration is at least 2 years. Its onset is usually early in adulthood, but recent evidence suggests that it may also arise later in life (NIH) and cause considerable morbidity. Dysthymia is a risk factor for major depression (NIH).
- *Adjustment disorder* with low mood is diagnosed when symptoms of low mood, often with anxiety, arise within 1 month of a major stressful event. The symptoms are insufficient for a particular diagnosis to be made in its own right (e.g. major depression) and resolution occurs within 6 months. Many cases of what were once termed 'neurotic depression' are encompassed by the term.

- Lastly, a new category of *vascular depression* has been proposed: the hypothesis is that damage to end-arteries supplying subcortical striato-pallido-thalamo-cortical pathways disrupts the neurotransmitter circuitry involved in mood regulation, and may thus cause or predispose to depression. The presumed basis, although unproven, is of vascular disease. Its features are listed in Box 3.3.

Box 3.3 Proposed features of vascular depression (Alexopoulos et al, 1997)

- Depression arises in later life
- Reduced depressive ideation
- Reduced insight
- Apathy and retardation
- Cognitive impairment (particularly executive dysfunction)
- Neurological evidence of ischaemic brain damage, notably affecting the white matter and subcortical areas

Summary of evidence

- A high proportion of clinically important depression in older people is non-major or subthreshold depression (IIa)
- For every case of major depression in later life there are between two and three non-major ones (minor or subthreshold depression) (IIa)
- Terms such as minor and subthreshold are increasingly used to refer to this type of depression, although it is likely to be a heterogeneous category (IIa)
- Such cases do not meet criteria for ICD or DSM major depression, although in reality they are clinically important (IIb)
- There is evidence that these non-major depressions (minor or subthreshold depressions) are nevertheless a significant cause of suffering and morbidity (IIa)

- There is also evidence that major and 'minor' depressions are on a continuum rather than quite separate disorders (IIa – extrapolated from mixed-aged populations)
- Minor (subthreshold) depression in older people is sometimes characterised by a distinct symptom profile which includes poor concentration and amotivation in association with poor health (IIa)
- Dysthymia is probably more common among older people than is realised, and is a risk factor for major depression (IIb)
- Another specific subtype occurs in patients who have late-onset depression with vascular disease and evidence on neuroimaging of subcortical white matter and gray matter changes – so-called 'vascular depression' (IIb)
- Bipolar disorder is uncommon in later life but associated with considerable morbidity (IIb)
- Organic causes of depressive episode occur more frequently in older than in younger patients (III)

Recommendations for practice

- In older people major depression, non-major depression and dysthymia are all targets for clinical intervention (B)
- Practitioners should be aware that subthreshold (minor) depression is a significant disorder and not a trivial one (B)
- It is important to have a high index of suspicion for subthreshold (minor) depression, particularly in people with poor health who have low mood, impaired cognition and low motivation (B)
- In older depressed people it is important to rule out organic causes (C)

Newer themes and issues for future research

- Whatever classification or name is used to delineate older people with non-major depression, it is likely that we are dealing with a heterogeneous group of mood disorders and that there are likely to be multiple aetiological pathways (WPA).
- In the search for subtypes, another distinction which is sometimes made is that of early- versus late-onset depression. However, the evidence seems to point towards different aetiological pathways, such as a greater likelihood of familial and developmental factors in early-onset patients, but with few differences in symptomatology (Brodaty et al, 2001).
- Vascular depression, as defined above, is associated with greater morbidity than non-vascular cases. This may be due to greater comorbidity, but also because of an associated dysexecutive syndrome, in itself disabling. This may arise because of damage to subcortical–frontal circuitry. There is also some evidence from case–control studies of a poorer response to treatment, especially single treatment with an antidepressant ('antidepressant monotherapy') (Simpson et al, 1997).
- As will be seen in Chapter 8, the best treatment for minor depression and dysthymia is not yet clear, largely because the necessary research has not been carried out. Ultimately, a useful classification of mood disorder would contain within it a treatment imperative; in other words, subtypes and categories would be linked to treatment indicators.

chapter 4

Prevalence of depressive disorder in later life

In the community

Studies from Europe and North America report a prevalence of major depression and (minor) subthreshold depression combined of between 8 and 15% (NIMH, PTD). In Europe the averaged prevalence was 12.3% (14.1% for women and 8.6% for men) (Copeland et al, 1999). In a meta-analysis of all reported studies worldwide it was 13.5% (Beekman et al, 1999). The ratio of major depression to (minor) subthreshold depression is approximately 3 : 1, although there was quite marked site variation in the European study. The prevalence and pattern is similar in North America.

As discussed earlier, these surveys identify older people with a depressive disorder serious enough to warrant intervention, whether they are classed as major, non-major (minor) depression or dysthymia.

In addition:

- Most studies of black and white elders in Britain and the United States find little difference in prevalence by race (Copeland et al, 1999).
- In some non-westernised societies the prevalence of depression has been reported as lower than in the west. An example is the Singaporean Chinese (Copeland et al, 1999).
- Some epidemiological studies adopt a hierarchical approach to diagnosing cases, meaning that a person may be classified as depressed or

demented but not both. The co-occurrence of depressive symptoms and cognitive impairment is common and increases exponentially with age. In one Finnish study the combination increased from 2% at age 65 to 24% at age 85 (Arve et al, 1999). It is therefore important to be aware of this, so that both disorders are managed.

There is an important ongoing debate about whether the prevalence of depressive disorder increases, remains static or even reduces with age – important not least because of the potential repercussions for resource allocation. Studies using criteria for major depressive episode have tended to show either static or decreased rates of depression with advancing age (Henderson et al, 1998), whereas those adopting broader criteria such as 'clinically relevant depression', or 'minor' depression, show rates that rise with age, either generally (Snowden, 2001) or specifically in women (Wu & Anthony, 2000). There are a number of explanations for this, ranging from differences in methods of ascertaining symptoms to differential symptom patterns with age. It is difficult to draw firm conclusions, but an overview of the literature suggests that it would be premature to assume that the prevalence of depression diminishes with age. It might be true that the prevalence of strictly defined major depression shows a decrease, but even if true this is more than offset by a high prevalence of subthreshold depression ('minor' depression).

In non-community settings

In addition to community (epidemiological) studies there have been a number of studies of the prevalence of depressive disorder among older people who attend primary care physicians, hospitals, or who are in nursing and residential care facilities. These studies are not as rigorous as the community ones, or have used widely differing measures, resulting in a much broader range in the prevalence figures. The following general observations can be made from a review of the literature:

- In older people who attend primary care physicians, significant depressive symptomatology has been reported in between 17 and 30% (PTD, NIH).
- Among hospitalised older patients the prevalence of depression ranges between 10 and 45% (PTD, NIH).
- In residential and nursing homes it is between 30 and 45% (PTD, NIH).
- A recent study from the United States found that approximately one in four patients who attended a geriatric emergency room had significant depression (Meldon et al, 1999).
- It has been reported that the rate of depressive disorder in older people who are in receipt of intensive home care support (probably a proxy measure of disability) is roughly double that of less frail individuals (Banerjee et al, 1996).

Figures such as these suggest an increasing prevalence of depression by dependency and/or disability. Chronicity of depressive symptoms may also be important. The prevalence of depression assessed cross-sectionally will be higher in populations where there is a high propor-

Summary of evidence

- Around one in every eight older people living in the community will have clinically important depressive symptoms, with women having higher rates then men (IIa)
- Although some societies report lower rates, the prevalence is remarkably consistent internationally (IIa)
- Among older people being attended by a primary care physician the prevalence is roughly doubled (IIa)
- Being in receipt of a high level of home support is associated with a rate of depression, about double that of less frail community-dwelling elders (IIa)
- Rates of depression are exceptionally high in hospitals and residential and nursing home facilities (IIa)

Recommendations for practice

- Depressive disorder, disability and dependency are all highly correlated. In general, the more disability the more depression. It is always worth considering depression in settings where disability is high, such as hospital wards, residential and nursing homes and the frail elderly at home (B)
- It is important to have a low threshold (high index of suspicion) for diagnosing depression in these settings, and also among patients consulting in primary care (B)

tion of patients with chronic symptoms, as opposed to short-lived and self-limiting ones.

Newer themes and issues for future research

- Although ethnic background and race have not proved to be major factors affecting prevalence, there may be complex interactions due to migration and acculturation. For example, among Mexican Americans, those with the least acculturation had the most depression (Gonzalez et al, 2001). In another study (Black et al, 1998) the effect of acculturation was modified by gender, with females being at increased risk. This is clearly an important avenue for future study.
- It is possible that the effect of low acculturation on depression rates is due to cultural barriers in getting help, but this requires further research.
- Paradoxically, in China there is emerging evidence that the prevalence of depression is higher in rural than in urban areas (WPA), whereas in some western societies the opposite has been found.

chapter 5

The aetiology of late-life depression

There are factors in a person's background that constitute a risk for depression and life events which often bring it about. Counterbalancing these are factors which are protective, sometimes called 'buffers'. Included here are psychosocial factors, such as social support and the security of the environment. It is usually the interplay of these that determines whether a person develops depressive disorder, rather than one particular factor. This is why some people develop depression even in the absence of an adverse life event, and why in others a major life event does not lead to depression. Lastly, the development of depressive disorder after a serious life event in an older person, such as a bereavement, does not make the depression 'understandable' and therefore not worth treating.

Importantly, there is no evidence (and perhaps indeed evidence to the contrary) that ageing *per se* is a risk factor for major depression. Associations that have been reported are usually explained by increased health difficulties, an important risk factor for depression, rather than age (PTD).

Risk factors for depressive disorder

Genetic susceptibility is substantially reduced in later-life depressive disorder compared to depression arising earlier in adulthood, particularly when onset is in later life (NIH, WPA, PTD).

Gender Females are most susceptible to depression. This does not appear to change significantly with age, although in the oldest old the ratio may reduce (NIH). Recent themes regarding why the risk in women is increased are discussed at the end of this chapter. Lastly, it has recently been suggested that gender may modify the effects of losses and transitions on triggering depression. In Hong Kong, Chou and Chi (2000) found that spousal bereavement in women led to an increase in depressive symptoms, whereas in men the moving out of children was associated with a decrease in depression.

A previous history of depressive disorder is an important predisposing factor to depression (PTD).

Civil status In cross-sectional studies widows, widowers and divorcees are more susceptible to depressive disorder (NIH, WPA, PTD).

Neurotransmitter changes Normal ageing is associated with decreased brain concentrations of serotonin, dopamine, noradrenaline and their metabolites, which would be expected to predispose to depression. However, the evidence is not consistent (PTD).

Neuroendocrine changes At all ages, depression is associated with hyperactivity and dysregulation of the hypothalamopituitary–adrenal (HPA) axis (NIH, PTD). Depressive disorder is associated with raised cortisol levels and cortisol non-suppression in response to exogenous steroids used to test the HPA axis, such as dexamethasone (NIH, PTD). However, similar changes may occur as part of the ageing process (PTD).

Structural brain changes Mild cerebral atrophy is present in depression at all ages, but whether it is a cause or consequence of depressive disorder is not clear. A recent focus of much research interest concerns the presence of deep white matter lesions and subcortical lesions in the gray matter which, thanks to new imaging techniques, have been shown to occur more commonly in major depressive disorder of late onset (PTD, WPA). These changes may be relevant to the well known finding that disorders which damage the subcortical–frontal circuitry of the brain are associated with a high incidence of depression. Examples include Huntington's disease, Parkinson's disease and some forms of stroke (Robinson et al, 1999). In addition, epidemiological databases, of which there are a number relating to older people, are beginning to shed light on potential causal mechanisms. For example, in one population-based study basal ganglia lesions were significantly associated with depressive symptoms in older people, whereas severity of white matter lesions were not (Steffens et al, 1999).

Vascular risk factors Epidemiological studies have highlighted an association between hypertension and depression. There is also recent evidence linking depression to a range of other vascular risk factors, including smoking and excessive consumption of alcohol in mixed age (Hamalainen et al, 2001) and older patients (Lyness et al, 1999a), and to some (but not all) serum lipids (Shibata et al, 1999). Interestingly, there is also evidence that low blood pressure is a risk factor for depressive disorder in older people (Stroup-Beham et al, 2000; Jorm, 2001). These have important implications for preventive care. Another factor, ε4 lipoprotein, which has been linked to vascular disease, was thought to be more common in patients with vascular depression, but recent data have not supported this.

Functional brain change Although it has been known for some time that blood perfusion is reduced in geriatric depression, recent data suggests that these findings do not necessarily normalise with treatment (Nobler et al, 1999), which would support the view that some patients with later-life major depression have irreversible brain changes.

Personality

- In clinical studies obsessional traits, 'avoidant' and 'dependent' personality types are overrepresented in older depressed patients (PTD).
- Those who have had a lifelong difficulty in forming close confiding relationships are also at risk (PTD).
- There is emerging evidence linking some personality traits (e.g. anxious, anankastic) to suicide (Harwood et al, 2001).

General health

- There is a strong association between depression and disability (the functional limitation arising from a disorder) due to medical conditions. In general, the greater the disability the more likely and/or more severe is depressive disorder (PTD, WPA).

- Another important concept is of handicap – the disadvantage in society that results from a disability. Recent research from the UK found handicap to be the most important predictor of new cases of depression in a community sample (Prince et al, 1998).

The relationship of depression to physical morbidity is covered in more detail in Chapter 6.

Being a carer of someone who is chronically ill is an important risk factor leading to depression. The association is particularly strong for dementia, and this has been demonstrated in a variety of different cultures (PTD).

Precipitating factors

Life events and stress Box 5.1 shows the common acute life events and the chronic social stressors that have been implicated in depression onset (PTD).

In a large epidemiological sample of people aged over 70 years, bereave-

Box 5.1 Aetiological stressful events in depressive disorder

Life events	Chronic stress
Bereavement	Declining health and mobility; dependence
Separation	Sensory loss, cognitive decline
Acute physical illness	Housing problems
Medical illness or threat to life of someone close	Major problems affecting family member
Sudden homelessness or having to move into an institution	Socioeconomic decline
Major financial crisis	Marital difficulties
Negative interactions with family member or friend	Problems at work; retirement
Loss of 'significant other' (including a pet)	Caring for a chronically ill and dependent family member
	Social isolation

ment by loss of spouse was associated with a ninefold increase in depressive disorder compared to those still married. Some widows and widowers experienced symptoms beyond 2 years. In this sample there was no association of depression with the expectedness or otherwise of the death (Turvey et al, 1999). In another study (van Grootheest et al, 1999) men adjusted less well after bereavement. The recently bereaved are therefore at high risk of depression and represent a group for whom screening would seem worthwhile.

Organic mood disorders due to drugs are not uncommon in older people. Box 5.2 lists drugs which at some time have been implicated in the literature, though often only in case reports. In practice, the most common offenders in contemporary practice are steroids, antihypertensives and analgesics, perhaps especially ones containing codeine (Romach et al, 1999).

In one cross-sectional study of mixed-age patients the medications most often associated with depression included calcium channel blockers, opiate analgesics and steroids, but not ACE inhibitors, lipid-lowering agents, β-blockers, digoxin or diuretics. In another large study tamoxifen given to women resident in nursing homes was associated with an increased rate of depression but a reduced rate of Alzheimer's disease (Breuer & Anderson, 2000). On the other hand, older women who take oestrogen-only preparations may be at reduced risk of depression (Whooley et al, 2000). Despite media interest, there is no evidence that exogenous androgens improve mood (NIH).

The true prevalence of depressive disorder caused or aggravated by medication is unknown, but almost certainly higher than supposed. It has been estimated that β-blockers alone could account for 1–10% of depressive disorders in older people (Dhondt & Hooijer, 1995). It is therefore important to keep an open mind about medication as a cause of depression.

Alcohol At any age, excessive consumption of alcohol can cause depression. Older people who start to drink excessively often experience isolation, loneliness, and may be suffering from depression. The prognosis for treating alcohol in this age group may be rather better than among those who drink from an early age (PTD).

Box 5.2 Centrally acting drugs that may cause or aggravate organic mood syndromes (PTD). Level IIb–III evidence

Central-acting drugs

Antihypertensive drugs

β-Blockers

Methyldopa

Reserpine

Clonidine

Calcium channel blockers (e.g. nifedipine)

Digoxin

Steroids

Analgesic drugs

Codeine

Opioids

Indomethacin

COX-2 inhibitors

Antiparkinson

L-Dopa

Amantadine

Tetrabenazine

Psychiatric drugs

Antipsychotics

Benzodiazepines

Buffering factors/protective (buffering) factors

Although much attention has been given to elucidating the risk factors and precipitating factors for depressive disorder, there are also factors, listed below, which may protect against it (PTD, NIH).

General medical care (evidence level III)

- Correcting physical deficits (e.g. sensory loss)
- Optimising general health
- Good nutrition
- Physical fitness

Coping behaviours (evidence level IIb)

- Adaptive, integrated personality
- Capacity for confiding relationships
- Active coping styles to overcome adversity (as opposed to helplessness).

Social supports (evidence level Ib)

- Adequate social network
- Tangible social support
- Positive perceptions of support
- Confiding relationships
- Religious/spiritual beliefs.

The relationship between social support and depressive disorder is complex. Social support appears to act as a buffer against depression or may ameliorate its impact. However, it is unclear whether it is the perception of the support received, the actual support received or some combination of the two; or whether the support ought to come from intimate others or from more diffuse relationships. However, both instrumental and emotional support appear to be important. Epidemiological data are shedding light on the complex interplay of risk factors. For example, in the Dutch AMSTEL study there was evidence that factors such as being married and having social support significantly reduced the negative impact of functional disability on the future of risk of developing depression (Schoevers et al, 2000). However, in a US study (Wallsten et al, 1999) the network had to be perceived by the older person as being helpful to their disability, otherwise tangible support had only a modest positive impact. Lastly, recently it has been shown that social support and the availability of a confiding relationship can offset the negative effect of disability (Schoevers et al, 2000).

Religious affiliation has generally been observed to have a protective effect on proneness to depression and survival generally in some cultures (Helm et al, 2000), although it may colour the presentation in other cultures (Braam et al, 2000).

Summary of evidence for causative factors in depression in later life

Predisposing factors

- Female gender (**IIa**)
- A prior history of depressive disorder (**IIa**)
- Widow/widowerhood; being divorced (**IIb**)
- Alteration in brain neuroamines and receptors (evidence mixed; not conclusive)
- Neuroendocrine disturbance (evidence mixed; not conclusive)
- Brain changes – mild atrophy; white matter and other changes; reduced perfusion ((**III**) associative findings; clear causal findings unproven)
- Personality – reduced capacity to form abiding attachments (**IIb**)
- Physical comorbidity; disability and handicap (**IIa**)
- Medication, alcohol and systemic disease (**IIa**)
- Care giving (**IIa**)
- Social disadvantage (**IIa**)
- Lack of social support (**IIa**)

Precipitating factors

- Adverse life events (**IIa**)
- Chronic stress (**IIb**)

Protective factors

- Optimal medical care (**III**)
- Positive coping style (**III**)
- Social support (**IIa**)

Recommendations for practice

- In practice it is important to take a multifactorial approach to causation in depression, recognising the roles of both individual susceptibility and adverse life events (B)
- Organic factors are often important in depressive disorder of older people; it is important to take a drug and alcohol history, including over-the-counter analgesics (B)
- Disability due to physical ill-health is strongly associated with depressive disorder; it should therefore be minimised as much as possible (B)
- Good medical care may reduce the incidence of depression or reduce its impact (C)
- The concept of handicap places disability in a social context. It is strongly associated with onset of depression, and much handicap can be prevented (B)
- Positive social and environmental factors (including the level and quality of support) may offset some of the negative effects of adverse life events and are important areas for intervention (B/C)

Newer themes and issues for future research

- There is some evidence that the gender difference may arise in part because women have a greater exposure to other risk factors for depression (Beekman et al, 1999).
- There is evidence from hospital-treated case series of hippocampal damage in late-life depression (Steffens et al, 2000). It is speculated that this arises from raised cortisol levels and may underpin the memory disorder which is often part of depressive disorder in later life.
- Perinatal susceptibility – recent evidence has shown that low birthweight is a risk factor for older men who develop depression

(Thompson et al, 2001a). Intriguingly, this suggests fetal undernutrition, perhaps leading to faulty development of the HPA axis.

- There is ongoing research exploring the relationship of depression in older people to the role of cytokines such as the interleukins in cortisol production, inflammation and immune system activation (NIH). More evidence is emerging of an association of interleukin-6, an inflammatory marker, with depressive disorder in later life. This suggests a possible immunoendocrine dysfunction (Dentino et al, 1999). This is an important area for future research.
- Interest remains in 'postmenopausal depression' – low mood, anxiety, fatigue, difficulty in making decisions and decreased libido – which, it is speculated, may be due to low levels of sex hormones, but this is very controversial (NIH).
- The relationship between abuse of elders, neglect and psychiatric disorder is beginning to be studied. In one study set in a geriatric clinic, patients referred because of these reasons had a higher rate of both depressive disorder and dementia than those referred for other reasons (Dyer et al, 2000).
- In depression among female patients of working age, 'fresh start' experiences, such as a new relationship, improve the outcome of depression, but there is no comparable research in older adults (Harris et al, 1999). This would be an important avenue to explore in older depressed people.

chapter 6

Comorbidity and depressive disorder

Comorbidity is the existence of separate conditions side by side. It is sometimes subdivided into physical comorbidity (due to coexisting physical disorders) and psychiatric comorbidity (when there are coexisting psychiatric symptoms or disorders).

Physical comorbidity

The interaction between ill-health and depressive disorders is complex and bidirectional. There has been a huge increase into research into comorbidity in recent years. The following is a summary of the recent literature.

- Depression is an independent risk factor for a number of conditions, including stroke – both in western (Jonas & Mussolino, 2000) and eastern (Ohira et al, 2001) cultures – and, in older people specifically, heart failure (Ariyo et al, 2000). There is even evidence of a link between chronic depression (of over 6 years' duration) in older people and the subsequent risk of developing a range of cancers (Penninx et al, 1998), although this effect was not observed in another study of women using a different instrument to measure depression (Whooley & Browner, 1999).
- Depressive symptoms (of all levels of severity, including mild ones)

add to disability from physical illness (Cronin-Stubbs et al, 2000). For example, in a community study of older Mexican Americans depression was associated with a greater health burden in persons with diabetes than in those free from diabetes. The burden was also greater in diabetic patients with depression than in those without (Black, 1999). This effect was evident even after controlling for the effects of sociodemographic variables, including immigrant status.

- Depressive symptoms are also associated with physical decline. In one study it was chronic rather than episodic depression that was independently associated with physical decline, highlighting the importance of prompt treatment of depression (Penninx et al, 2000).
- Depression worsens the prognosis for a coexisting physical disorder, such as myocardial infarction (NIH).
- Depressive symptoms in men aged over 75 are associated with a greater than threefold increase in subsequent hospitalisation for a medical disorder (Huang et al, 2000).
- Disability is a risk factor for depression (Lenze et al, 2001b).
- Sensory impairment – hearing and visual impairment – is associated with depression (PTD).
- Chronic ill-health contributes to a poor prognosis in depressive disorders (PTD).
- Nutritional status can both affect and be affected by depression (PTD).
- In a model based on a large community sample, depression fitted best as a mediator between general health perceptions and overall quality of life (Sullivan et al, 2000).

Because of these interactions the whole person must be considered. Evidence from primary care has suggested that practitioners often adopt an ‘either/or’ approach to their patients, tending to focus either on the physical disorder or the psychiatric symptoms, when attention to both is required (PTD).

Hypochondriasis

This is briefly mentioned as it is such a frequent symptom in older people. An excessive preoccupation with bodily health and bodily function may be associated with physiological changes due to ageing or disease, with physical disease in peers or peer expectations (for example concerning the regularity of bowel habit), or with depressive disorder.

Pain

This too is common in older people. Depressive disorder alters the pain threshold – a pain once tolerated may become unbearable when the person becomes depressed. In a recent study from China there was a strong association between depression and headache (Wang et al, 1999), suggesting an interaction between the two.

Organic depressive disorder

As already discussed, the term organic depressive disorder means that the depressive state has arisen because of a pathophysiological link between the underlying physical condition and depression. The conditions listed in Box 6.1 are those for which a causative link has been proposed. Unfortunately, the level of evidence varies from rigorous data obtained from large populations to case reports.

Common medical conditions which are often associated with depression

There are a number of conditions which affect older people in particular and which have been linked to a high rate of depressive disorder. Box 6.2 lists those for which there is a good body of evidence in older people. Their presence should alert the clinician to think about whether a depressive disorder could be present alongside the medical condition. There is overlap between Boxes 6.1 and 6.2 because in practice causation is often multifactorial. For example, in Parkinson's disease a link between depression and depleted serotoninergic metabolites has been proposed (suggesting an organic mood disorder), but depressive symptoms also occur at times when the patient's physical condition alters suddenly (implying psychological factors in causation).

Box 6.1 Causes of organic mood disorder (evidence levels IIB–IV)

Endocrine/metabolic
Hypo/hyperthyroidism
Cushing's disease
Hypercalcaemia (primary hyperparathyroidism or carcinoma)
Pernicious anaemia

Organic brain disease
Cerebrovascular disease/stroke
CNS tumours
Parkinson's disease
Alzheimer's disease
Systemic lupus erythematosus

Occult carcinoma
Pancreas
Lung

Chronic infections
Neurosyphilis
Brucellosis
Neurocysticercosis

Box 6.2 Some of the common medical conditions in older people which are associated with a high prevalence of depressive disorder (NIH, PTD, WPA)

- Cancer
- Stroke
- Parkinson's disease
- Hip fracture
- Myocardial infarction and heart failure
- Chronic obstructive pulmonary disease and asthma

In the conditions listed in the Box 6.2 the point-prevalence of depressive symptoms is up to 40% for some conditions, although the rate of major depression is considerably lower (5–10%); this is still higher than among healthy older people living at home.

As discussed, in a number of these conditions there is a two-way causative process. For example, patients who have had a stroke, hip fracture (Holmes & House, 2000), myocardial infarction or heart failure have a high incidence of depression, but depressive disorder is independently associated with a higher than expected rate of stroke and cardiovascular disease, including cardiovascular mortality; also, recent evidence has suggested that for women aged over 50 being depressed is associated with a higher than expected rate of hip fracture, even allowing for prescribed medication (Forsen et al, 1999). Having a serious adverse life event before a stroke can also markedly increase the incidence of depression after it (Bush, 1999).

Lastly, until recently it was thought that stroke patients with a lesion close to the anterior pole of the left hemisphere were especially prone to depression but recent evidence does not suggest such a specific association (Carson et al, 2000) – all stroke patients are at risk.

Psychiatric comorbidity

'Neurotic' symptoms

Unlike in younger people, depressive disorder in older people is less likely to be associated with another major psychiatric diagnosis, such as personality disorder or substance misuse. Similarly, the so-called neurotic symptoms (anxiety, obsessive–compulsive disorder, panic and hysteria) are uncommon as primary diagnoses in older adults. Usually, when they occur for the first time in an older person they suggest an underlying depressive disorder which they may easily mask. An exception may be phobic disorder. Community studies from North America and England have shown it to be quite common, especially situational phobia. An example would be of an older person recovering from a fall who develops agoraphobic symptoms in relation to crossing a large open space such as a shopping mall.

Likewise, case-level symptoms of anxiety affect upward of 5% of older people, although generalised anxiety disorder remains highly correlated with depression, even in the very old (Forsell & Winblad, 1998). When anxiety and depression occur together it seems that benzodiazepines rather than antidepressants are prescribed (NIH, PTD). Detection of underlying depression is therefore important.

Although earlier it was stated that marked anxiety can mask depression in older people, in one survey of primary care physicians the symptom of anxiety was regarded as such a strong indicator of psychiatric disorder that, paradoxically, it led to the 'unmasking' of the depression (Kirby et al, 1999b). Whether this is true in everyday practice is not known.

Dementia

Both anxiety and depressive symptoms are common in dementia. Unfortunately, because of the use of different measures in research, rates reportedly vary from 0 to 85%. Using a weighted average, Allen and Burns (1995) calculated a prevalence of moderate to severe depressive disorder in patients with Alzheimer's disease of 20% – higher than in aged-matched community residents. Also, the literature has consistently reported that depression is more common in vascular as opposed to Alzheimer-type dementia (Allen & Burns, 1995). Depression in dementia has been shown to accelerate functional decline (Ritchie et al, 1998). Lastly, it is worth restating that caregivers of those with dementia have high levels of depression.

Summary of evidence

- Depression in older people often coexists with other psychiatric symptoms, such as anxiety (IIa)
- Dementia is associated with a high rate of comorbid depression (IIa)
- Frailty, disability and dependency are highly correlated with depressive disorder in older people (Ib)

- Some physical disorders may predispose to or cause depression. Those most frequently encountered are stroke, Parkinson's disease, hip fracture, cancer, myocardial infarction, heart failure and chronic pulmonary disease (IIa)
- For stroke and heart disease, and perhaps cancer and hip fracture, there is evidence that depressive disorder itself predisposes to these conditions (IIa)
- In practice physicians tend to focus on either the physical or the mental, and not both (IIb)
- Some physical disorders seem able to precipitate depression via a direct effect on the brain neurotransmitter systems, such as serotonin (IIb)
- Other disorders exert an effect through a more complex interplay of physical, psychological and social factors (IIa)

Recommendations for practice

- In order to achieve optimal outcomes for the patient both mental and physical health problems should be treated together, as the prognosis of the one is closely associated with that of the other (A)
- In dementia it is important to check for signs and symptoms of depression, as this is common (B)
- It is important to check for signs and symptoms of depression in patients with Parkinson's disease, heart disease, chronic pulmonary disease, or who have had a stroke or hip fracture, as they are at high risk (B)
- It is worth asking the patient about adverse life events prior to a serious medical illness, as this may have been involved in causing depression and may require intervention in its own right (for example bereavement counselling) (C)

Newer themes and issues for future research

- Subcortical brain dysfunction may be the common link in the genesis of depressive disorder arising in degenerative brain diseases such as Parkinson's and Huntington's disease (Robinson et al, 1999).
- Depression may an independent risk factor for disorders such as cancer, probably through an effect on the immune system; but this requires further research (Dentino et al, 1999).
- Strong associations are reported for depression and heart disease, illustrating how important it is to treat both (Ariyo et al, 2000; Abramson et al, 2001). The benefits of treating comorbid depression in heart disease are being reported in younger adults, and data will hopefully follow for older patients too.

chapter 7

Assessment

Screening

Screening should be considered as part of an overall detection and management strategy.

The two most widely used scales are the Geriatric Depression Scale (GDS) and the Center for Epidemiological Studies Depression scale (CES-D). The latter, as its name suggests, has been used throughout the world as a screening instrument to identify depressive disorder in epidemiological samples. It is used rather less as a clinical tool. There are concerns that its properties may be affected by local culture (Mackinnon et al, 1998; Cole et al, 2000) and that it has too many somatic items (Katona & Livingston, 2000). It will not therefore be discussed further.

The GDS was published in 1983 as a 30-item self-rated questionnaire (Yesavage et al, 1983), although it is more often used with assistance, which does not appear to adversely affect its properties. For probable caseness the cut-off is 11 and above. In 1986 a 15 item version was introduced (Appendix G). The most appropriate cut-off will depend on the aims of its use. A cut-off of 4/5 produces very high sensitivity (90% or better) but low (of the order of 65%) specificity, meaning that quite a lot of people screened positive will prove not to have depressive disorder. With a cut-off of 6/7 the sensitivity falls to about 80% but the specificity increases to around 80%, meaning that some patients who screened negatively will nevertheless have depression. A cut-off of

5/6 gives intermediate results (Almeida & Almeida, 1999). It performs satisfactorily in patients with mild to moderate dementia but not with severe dementia. Recently a 12-item version has been introduced for use in residential and care homes which was not affected by moderate to high levels of cognitive impairment (Sutcliffe et al, 2000). A shorter version has been developed and validated for visually impaired older people (Galaria et al, 2000). In this version, endorsing any two of the following: dissatisfaction with life; feeling helpless; reporting problems with memory; and lost activities and interests; yielded a sensitivity of 0.71 and a specificity of 0.88.

The GDS has been translated in many countries, from China to Chile. It has good cross-cultural validity (Rait et al, 1999). As such it is the recommended scale for detecting depression, with the 15-item version accruing most evidence. There is a website for the GDS which details current versions and translations (http://stanford.edu/~yesavage/GDS.html).

There are also four-, five- and 10-item versions of the GDS. In the four-item version the questions are: Are you basically satisfied with your life? Do you feel that your life is empty? Are you afraid that something bad is going to happen to you? Do you feel happy most of the time? Endorsing any two or more of these signifies probable depression. There is even a single-item version, but doubts have been cast over its validity and reliability (Almeida & Almeida, 1999). The four-item GDS is recommended only for rapid screening. A five-item version has been developed which has demonstrated a sensitivity of almost 100% and a specificity of 85% in geriatric outpatients (Hoyl et al, 1999).

The Cornell Scale for Depression in Dementia (Alexopoulos et al, 1988) takes a different approach by synthesising questions derived from an informant and by observation. Its 19 items cover anxiety, sadness, lack of reactivity to pleasant events, irritability, agitation, retardation, multiple physical complaints, loss of interests, appetite loss, weight loss, lack of energy, diurnal variation, difficulty falling asleep, multiple awakenings during sleep, early-morning wakening, suicidal wishes or intent, self-depreciation, pessimism and mood-congruent delusions. Each item is rated on a three-point scale. There may be several iterations as the rater seeks concordance between the caregiver's description and the observations of the patient, so that the internal validity and reliability are good. It takes about 30 minutes to administer and is not therefore an ideal tool for primary care.

EASYcare has arisen from a European collaborative venture and a brief six-item cognitive screening questionnaire (Katzman et al, 1983) which is reproduced in Appendix D. It is a geriatric assessment tool which incorporates the GDS-4 and a brief six-item cognitive screening questionnaire. It has been piloted in 18 European countries and details can be found on the website: http://www.shef.ac.uk/sisa/easycare/index.shtml.

BASDEC (Brief Assessment Depression Schedule Cards) was developed to aid the detection of depressive disorder in medically ill patients. It comprises 19 questions, several of which are similar to the GDS but printed on cards. The patient has to point his or her response to a 'yes' or 'no' card. It is useful in situations where privacy is at a premium and it has been translated into a number of Asian languages. BASDEC has been used effectively in recent research on older patients with Chronic Obstructive Pulmonary Disease (Yohanness et al, 2000).

No screening questionnaire should be used in isolation. First, no version has 100% sensitivity and 100% specificity. In other words, they are not a substitute for clinical evaluation. A positive test merely indicates a need for a full evaluation (Katona & Livingston, 2000). Secondly, the use of questionnaires without adequate support in primary care has not led to improvements in care delivered (Katona & Livingston, 2000).

Summary of evidence – screening questionnaires for depressive disorder in older people (evidence level Ib–IIb)

- GDS (4-, 5-, 10-, 12-, 15- and 30-item versions)
- Cornell Scale for Depression in Dementia
- BASDEC
- EASYcare

Screening programmes are most *efficient* when targeted at high-risk populations, such as those listed below and are most *effective* when combined with agreed management protocols (PTD, NIH).

Recommendations for targeted screening in primary care (PTD, NIH): level B

- Recent major physical illness (within 3 months)
- Chronic handicapping illness
- Receiving high level of home support (personal care)
- Recent bereavement (3–6 months)
- Socially isolated older people
- Those who persistently complain of loneliness
- Patients with persistent sleep difficulties

Clinical evaluation

There are five components that the clinician assessing the patient should address. These are listed in Box 7.1 and amplified below. However, practitioners can enhance their chances of successfully detecting depressive disorder in an older person by attending to the points raised in Box 7.2 (PTD).

The following points are designed to help the practitioner to be comprehensive in his or her assessment:

- History (core symptoms; onset of depression; triggers; previous history of depression; previous treatments for depression; factors which may maintain or potentiate depression; up-to-date list of

Box 7.1 Aspects of the clinical evaluation of an older person presenting with depression

- History
- Mental state
- Risk assessment
- Physical examination
- Physical investigation

Box 7.2 Strategies which are more likely to lead to positive identification of depressive disorder in older people

- Become familiar with the cores symptoms of depressive disorders
- Maintain awareness of the high frequency of depressive disorders
- Know in what ways ageing may alter the presentation of depression in older adults
- Give equal attention to physical and mental health
- Develop skills for clinical interviewing of older people
- Remember that a significant life event can trigger a real depressive disorder
- Avoid therapeutic nihilism ('nothing works')
- Remember that depressive disorders are not a normal part of ageing

Taken from WPA International Committee for Prevention and Treatment of Depression. *Depressive Disorders in Older Persons* NCM Publishers Inc, NY (referenced as PTD)

medications; evidence of alcohol or tranquilliser misuse). Speaking to someone close to the patient will usually clarify aspects of the history and is recommended.

- Mental state (evidence of psychotic symptoms, suicidality or cognitive impairment – use of relevant screen, such as the Mini-Mental State Examination recommended – Folstein et al, 1975).
- Risk assessment for suicide and depression-induced self-neglect should be conducted in all cases where depression has been diagnosed. Most cases of completed suicide have consulted a primary care doctor within the month preceding the act (PTD, WPA; see also Chapter 9).
- Physical examination, including focused neurological examination (to identify organic causes of depression; to identify any contraindications to particular classes of antidepressants).

- Physical investigations (to identify an organic cause for depression; Box 7.3). It is recommended that patients with depressive disorder should receive the following tests (PTD, EXP): blood count, serum chemistry for renal function, liver enzymes, glucose and calcium, B_{12}, serum and red cell folate, and thyroid function tests. In addition, other non-routine tests such as syphilis serology, a chest X-ray, brain scan electroencephalogram (EEG) or ECG may be requested, depending on clinical findings.

Box 7.3 Laboratory and other investigations in later-life depression

Investigation	*Routine*
Full blood count	Yes
Serum chemistry	Yes
Serum glucose	Yes
Liver enzymes	Yes
Calcium	Yes
Thyroid function	Yes
B_{12}	Yes
Folate	Yes
Syphilitic serology	Only if indicated by history or physical findings
Chest X-ray	Only if indicated by history or physical findings
Electrocardiogram (ECG/EKG)	Only if indicated by history, and/or prior to commencement of some antidepressants (e.g. older tricyclics)
Brain scan	Only if clinically indicated
EEG	Only if clinically indicated

Rating scales

For a list of scales, see Burns et al, 1999.

The use of a cognitive screening examination for dementia is recommended (EXP). A widely used scale is the Mini-Mental Status Examination (MMSE) (Folstein et al, 1975). However, the MMSE can take 10–15 minutes to administer so that shorter scales may be more useful in the primary care setting in particular. An example is that of Katzman et al (1983), Appendix D as mentioned. Self-rated scales for detecting depression may be used, such as the Geriatric Depression Rating Scale, which is reproduced in Appendix G.

The Cornell Scale for Depression in Dementia is an interviewer-rated instrument which can assist in detecting depression in comorbid dementia. This has been discussed.

Lastly, there are interviewer-rated instruments able to measure severity of depression which can assist in monitoring response to treatment. Two that have been validated for use in older people (Mottram et al, 2000) are the Hamilton Rating Scale for Depression (Hamilton, 1960) and the Montgomery–Asberg Depression Rating Scale (Montgomery and Asberg, 1979). These are reproduced in Appendices E and F. Neither scale is a screening instrument for depression, but patients with moderate depressive episode generally score 18 or more on the Hamilton and 20 or above on the Montgomery–Asberg scale.

In primary care time is at a premium. Nevertheless, when it comes to making treatment decisions, especially whether or not to change therapy (Chapter 8), severity scales can be very helpful by adding objectivity to the assessment.

Risk assessment

Predicting suicide is imprecise, as many more depressed individuals experience thoughts that life is not worth living than ever attempt suicide. However, in developed societies it is older people who are most at risk of suicide, and about three-quarters of older people with depression who kill themselves will have had recent contact with their primary care physician (NIH, PTD). The following indicate higher risk (EXP):

- *Demography* Older age (especially those over 80), isolation and male gender
- *History* A history of previous attempt(s); evidence of planning, such as altering wills; a recent bereavement
- *Physical factors* Chronic and painful medical disorder; alcohol misuse; abuse of sedatives/hypnotics
- *Mental state* Suicidal thoughts; plans of suicide; marked agitation (patient is objectively restless, and also has an inner sense of restlessness for much of the time); profound hopelessness, feelings of worthlessness, guilt or self-reproach; marked insomnia; marked hypochondriasis; psychotic ideation.

Summary of evidence

- Clinical knowledge, appropriate attitudes to older people and good interview skills will lessen the chances of overlooking depressive disorder (IV)
- A diagnosis of depressive disorder is the leading risk factor for suicide in older people (IIa)
- A comprehensive assessment of depressive disorder in an older person includes taking a history, performing an assessment of the mental state and of risk, carrying out a relevant physical examination, and requesting a range of appropriate tests (IV)
- The investigations most relevant are a blood count, serum chemistry, thyroid function, B_{12} and folate (IV)
- Those most at risk of suicide are isolated men aged over 80 with a previous history of attempting self-harm; those who have chronic often painful conditions or who abuse alcohol or pills; or who have a clinical picture of severe depression (III)
- Most older people who have killed themselves have seen their primary care physician within the preceding month (IIa)
- There are a number of reliable instruments which can be used to rate depressive symptoms (Ib)

Recommendations for practice

The recommendations constitute Category D evidence. This is an area where practice is informed as much by experience as by research. Current best practice regarding assessment of the older person is that the following should be conducted on patients presenting with depressive disorder:

- History
- Mental state
- Risk assessment for suicide and non-deliberate self-harm
- Focused physical and neurological examination
- Investigations: blood count, serum chemistry, thyroid function, B_{12} and folate, with other tests as indicated
- Patients at high risk of suicide should be referred to specialist psychiatric services without delay
- In addition, it is recommended that a rating scale be used such as the Hamilton Rating Scale for Depression or the Montgomery–Asberg Depression Rating Scale be used to assess response to treatment.

Another way in which older people place themselves at risk of harm is by self-neglect. Whether or not this can be construed as a form of attempted suicide is a matter of debate. Nevertheless, older people become physically compromised much more quickly than do younger adults, so the consequences of dietary neglect, neglect of heating etc. can rapidly place the individual at great risk, whether intended or not.

Newer themes and issues for future research

The aim of a large initiative in the United States, PROSPECT, is to help equip primary care physicians with the skills to detect and manage depression, in the expectation that this will, in time, reduce suicide rates (Brown et al, 2001). The results of this trial, when published, will enable further refinements of guidelines.

chapter 8

Management

General principles

Ideally, the management of depressive disorder in older people is multimodal (involving physical and psychological modalities along with social interventions) and multidisciplinary (with help from specialists such as nurses, social workers and occupational therapists and, as needed, from dietitians, speech and language therapists and podiatrists). The goals of treatment of a depressive episode are:

- To bring about a remission of *all* depressive symptoms. Residual symptoms increase the risk of chronic depression, impair recovery in physical illness and predispose to physical illness (NIH, EXP, Keller & Boland, 1998)
- Risk reduction – of suicide or harm from self-neglect (PTD, NIH)
- To help the patient achieve optimal function, both physically and socially (PTD, WPA)
- To treat the whole person, including physical health, nutrition, poor mobility and contextual issues, such as reduced social support (PTD, NIH)
- To prevent relapse and recurrence (PTD, NIH, EXP).

Ways to achieve these goals (Box 8.1) include:

- A risk assessment and the monitoring of risk (by ensuring regular review of the patient) (PTD)

Box 8.1 Some management goals and how to achieve them

Goal	Ways to achieve goals
Risk reduction – of suicide or harm from self-neglect	A risk assessment and monitoring of risk Prompt referral of urgent cases to a specialist
Remission of all depressive symptoms	Providing appropriate treatment (usually with an antidepressant and/or a psychological treatment) Giving the patient and his/her supporters timely education about depression and its treatment
To help the patient achieve optimal function	Enable practical support Ensure access to appropriate agencies which can help
To treat the whole person, including somatic problems	Treat coexisting physical health problems Reduce wherever possible the effects of handicap caused by factors such as chronic disease, sensory impairment and poor mobility Review medication and withdraw unnecessary ones
To prevent relapse and recurrence	Educate the patient about staying on medication once recovered Continuing treatment for 12 months after recovery (see Chapter 10) Give maintenance treatment (preventive treatment) when indicated (see Chapter 10)

- Providing education about depressive disorder for the patient and his/her supporters (PTD)
- Treating coexisting physical health problems (PTD, NIH)
- Reducing wherever possible the effects of handicap caused by factors such as chronic disease, sensory impairment and poor mobility (PTD, NIH)
- Attending to social care needs (especially loneliness and social isolation) (PTD)
- Reviewing medication and discontinuing unnecessary prescriptions. For example, in a recent study codeine, a drug commonly used in over-the-counter prescriptions, was significantly associated with depression (Romach et al, 1999). This may be because it is a causal agent or because it is used by depressed persons as self-medication
- Intervene with appropriate treatment; initially this will be either an antidepressant and/or a psychological intervention (BAP)
- Prompt referral of patients who require specialist old age psychiatric services; the main indicators are (BAP, EXP):
  - Suicide risk
  - Harm from self-neglect
  - The diagnosis is uncertain or unclear
  - The diagnosis is of bipolar disorder
  - Complex case (e.g. multiple physical problems)
  - No or only partial response to two treatment trials. However, the practitioner may consider seeking help if a single trial of an antidepressant given in adequate dosage for sufficient time (see below) has failed
  - Presence of psychotic symptoms.

It is recommended (Box 8.2) that a plan of management be agreed with the patient and, where relevant, his or her caregiver(s) to outline the goals, when they are to be reviewed, what treatment modalities are to be recommended and who will implement them (PTD).

The modern management of depressive disorder is divided into three phases (PTD, NIH, WPA, EXP). These are:

Box 8.2 Planning care

- Outline goals of treatment
- Say when they will be reviewed
- Specify treatment modalities
- Say who will be involved in implementing the plan

- Acute treatment phase – to bring about recovery and remission of symptoms (a remission)
- Continuation phase – to prevent the same episode of illness returning (a relapse)
- Maintenance (or prophylaxis) phase – to prevent a future episode (a recurrence).

A patient may show a response but still have symptoms. Remission is the point at which all or almost all symptoms have disappeared. The period denoted by continuation therapy is defined by consensus. In younger patients it is set at 6 months, but in older patients the period of continuation after major depression will usually last between 12 and 24 months (NIH, EXP); see also Chapter 10.

Acute treatment phase

Box 8.3 outlines the types of intervention, along with the level of evidence, for treatments which are regularly used or have been proposed for depressive disorder in older adults.

It is reassuring to have such a wide range of treatments and treatment modalities, but the evidence base for some is sparse, although this does not mean that they are not effective. In determining the most appropriate treatment it is first necessary to characterise the type of depression (Box 8.4). Based on current evidence, the following guidance is offered (BAP, EXP):

- For *psychotic depression* a specialist should be consulted. Although the evidence is not in complete agreement much of it suggests that an

Box 8.3 Treatment modalities in depressive disorder (WPA, EXP)

Psychoeducation (IIa)

Physical treatments

- Antidepressant drugs (Ia)
- Electroconvulsive therapy (ECT) (Ia)
- Transcranial magnetic stimulation (TMS) (III)
- Vagal nerve stimulation (VNS) (no evidence in elderly)

Psychological treatments

- Supportive (III)
- Cognitive behaviour therapy (CBT) (Ia)
- Interpersonal therapy (IPT) (Ia)
- Problem-solving therapy (IIb)
- Family therapy (III)
- Psychodynamic psychotherapy (Ib)
- Self-help (IIb)

Other

- Light (photo)therapy (IIb)
- Exercise (III)
- Music therapy (III)
- Herbal (St John's Wort) (no evidence in elderly)

antidepressant alone will be insufficient to bring about recovery, and that often ECT will be needed, or a combination of an antidepressant and an antipsychotic.

- For *severe (non-psychotic) depression* antidepressant treatment combined wherever possible with a psychotherapeutic intervention should be the first line. Sometimes ECT is recommended (see below). Treatment will be indicated irrespective of whether there is a clear precipitant for the depression, or whether there is a physical disorder present, although the latter may influence the choice of treatment.

- For *moderate depression* antidepressants are again the first line of treatment. However, where resources permit or the patient expresses a preference, then psychological treatments (CBT, problem-solving therapy or IPT, with some evidence for brief psychodynamic psychotherapy) are effective.
- For *dysthymia* there is evidence from mixed-age patients (BAP) and in one trial of older patients in primary care (who had a minimum or three or four symptoms from Box 1.1) that antidepressants should be used in preference to psychological treatment as first-line treatment (Williams et al, 2000).
- For *subthreshold (minor) depression of recent onset* (approximately 1–3 weeks):
  - There is no evidence that antidepressants are effective.
  - The recommended approach is to offer education and support to the patient – 'watchful waiting' (BAP, EXP).
- For more *persistent subthreshold depression* ('minor' depression lasting 4 weeks or longer) there is emerging evidence that an antidepressant may be more effective than a placebo (Williams et al, 2000). In persistent cases of this kind it is good practice to offer the patient a therapeutic trial of an antidepressant.
- The differentiation of *grief* from depressive disorder can be difficult. In the early stages of a bereavement a high percentage of patients have symptoms similar to those of major depression. When should these symptoms be treated? In the initial weeks support rather than drugs should be offered. The main indications for a trial of an antidepressant are:
  - Duration: the most severe symptoms will have improved after 6 months (although some symptoms may remain for up to 2 years)
  - Intensity: suicidal thoughts, a profound wish to join the one mourned, pervasive guilt (not merely self-recrimination for not having done more to prevent death), retardation and 'mummification' (maintaining grief by keeping everything unchanged) are all pointers to medical intervention, similar to that for moderate-to-severe major depression.

Box 8.4 Summary of evidence – treatment modality and type of depression (evidence levels Ia–IIa)

Type of depression	Treatment modality
Psychotic depression	Combined antidepressant or ECT – urgent referral indicated
Severe (non-psychotic depression)	Combined antidepressant and psychological therapy
Moderate depressive episode	Antidepressant *or* psychological therapy (CBT, problem-solving, IPT or brief psychodynamic psychotherapy)
Dysthymia	Antidepressant
Recent-onset subthreshold (minor) depression	Watchful waiting
Persistent subthreshold (minor) depression	Antidepressant
Grief/bereavement	Treat as for moderate depression if duration and intensity indicate help needed

Physical treatments – antidepressants

Box 8.5 lists by class the currently available antidepressants used to treat older people. However, before initiating treatment it is important to offer appropriate education.

Initiating antidepressants – what to tell the patient

Involving the patient by giving education about antidepressant treatment improves compliance (PTD). Education may cover the following:

- Counselling the patient that depression is a treatable disorder

Box 8.5 Main antidepressants by class

- Older tricyclics
  - Amitriptyline
  - Imipramine
  - Nortriptyline
  - Dosulepin (dothiepin)
- Newer tricyclics
  - Lofepramine
- Selective serotonin reuptake inhibitors (SSRI)
  - Fluvoxamine
  - Fluoxetine
  - Paroxetine
  - Sertraline
  - Citalopram
- Other antidepressants
  - Nefazodone ($5HT_2$ antagonist)
  - Trazodone
  - Mianserin
- Non-reversible inhibitor of monoamine oxidase inhibitors (MAOI)
  - Phenelzine
- Reversible inhibitor of monoamine oxidase A (RIMA)
  - Moclobemide
- Serotonin and noradrenaline reuptake inhibitors (SNRI)
  - Venlafaxine
  - Milnacipran
- Noradrenaline reuptake inhibitor (NaRI)
  - Reboxetine
- Noradrenergic and selective serotonin antidepressants (NaSSA)
  - Mirtazepine
- Others
  - Bupropion
  - Alprazolam (long-acting benzodiazepine)
  - Methylphenidate
  - Tianeptine

- Explaining that antidepressants are non-addictive
- Discussing the importance of compliance (taking tablets regularly, not missing tablets, no sudden discontinuation)
- Evidence from mixed-age study populations suggests that giving a leaflet is less effective than medication counselling delivered either face-to-face or over the telephone. Although some training is required, this may be given by a member of the primary care team
- Counsel the patient not to stop treatment when recovery has occurred.

It is not intended to cover in detail all the antidepressants listed in Box 8.5. For instance, non-reversible MAOIs are of proven efficacy in older people, but their adverse effects on blood pressure and the need for dietary restrictions mean that they are seldom a first choice nowadays for the older primary care patient. Likewise, the evidence regarding drugs such as alprazolam and methylphenidate is limited in older ambulatory patients (McCusker et al, 1998), and they are not recommended in primary care management. In the UK buproprion is only licensed for smoking cessation, but is used quite extensively in slow-release form in North America (Steffens et al, 2001; EXP). Reboxetine, a specific norepinephrine (noradrenaline) reuptake inhibitor, is not recommended for use in older people in the UK because of a lack of data, although there are some safety data and uncontrolled efficacy data in the elderly (Andreoli et al, 1999; Aguglia, 2000). In France a trial of tianeptine in primary care patients showed it to be considerably less effective than fluoxetine (Guelfi et al, 1999). Milnacipran, a combined reuptake inhibitor, is used in continental Europe, but there are few data regarding the elderly.

In practice, the two most frequently prescribed classes are the tricyclics and the SSRIs. In the US expert panel report (EXP) the majority of those surveyed would avoid tertiary tricyclics (amitriptyline, imipramine, doxepin) in older people.

Pharmacokinetics

Older people have marked interindividual variability in how they metabolise drugs. For many of the older tricyclics this means it is difficult to predict the target dose. The adage 'start low, go slow' then applies. This is less of a problem with the newer drugs, for which the starting dose and the therapeutic dose are identical. However, many therapeutic trials have excluded the very old and the very frail, so that our knowledge of the properties of the newer drugs is not complete (WPA). It is therefore advisable to 'start low, go slow' (PTD) in patients who are frail (for example, starting with half dosages of the SSRIs and building up over 4–7 days). Box 8.6 provides information on starting dosages (EXP).

Efficacy

A number of reviews and meta-analyses exist demonstrating the superiority of antidepressant drugs over placebo for major depression. There is good evidence of their efficacy in older patients too. For example, Mittmann et al (1997) conducted a wide-ranging meta-analysis of antidepressants used to treat depression in older people, who they defined as being aged over 60. There were no significant differences in efficacy between any class of antidepressant. The response rates were approximately 30% to placebo and 60% to active drug. Although these are similar to rates reported in the literature in younger people, in another meta-analysis the response rate to active drug was only 50% (Gerson et al, 1999). Interestingly, there were no differences in tolerability or side effects in either meta-analysis, although similar studies of mixed-age patients (BAP) have found small but significant advantages in favour of newer antidepressants, particularly over the older tricyclics. A Cochrane evidence-based review of the literature examining only studies in which there was a placebo arm also found no differences in efficacy of older and newer antidepressants (Wilson et al, 2001). The number needed to treat to prevent one bad outcome (NNT) for the antidepressants that have been studied the most, the tricyclics, was four. This figure is equal to or better than many other treatments in medicine. For the SSRIs the NNT was lower, at 7 : 1, although the methodology only included two trials, both of fluoxetine. For minor depression and dysthymia there is limited evidence of efficacy of antidepressants. In the only adequately designed study to date (Williams et al, 2000), patients in primary care with either minor depression or dysthymia, but with duration of at least

4 weeks and three to four symptoms of depression (Box 1.1), paroxetine treatment was significantly more effective than placebo for dysthymia and modestly more effective than placebo for minor depression. The main deficiency in all the trial data is the small numbers included of the oldest-old and of those with marked frailty.

In addition, the following are important:

- In primary care there is evidence that older antidepressants are less likely to be prescribed in adequate dosage than newer agents. For example, a large survey from Nova Scotia in the mid-1990s showed that the SSRIs, secondary amine tricyclics and tertiary amine tricyclics the proportions deemed by an expert panel to be an adequate dosage were 79%, 45% and 31%, respectively (Rojas-Fernandez et al, 1999). Encouragingly, in the above study there was a downward trend in the inappropriate use of antidepressants given to older people, from two-thirds to just over a half, but these figures are still a cause for concern.
- In the UK there is evidence that benzodiazepines are more likely to be prescribed than antidepressants (which were only given to 10% of those diagnosed with depression in one study – Wilson et al, 1999).
- Some advice (PTD) recommends that primary care prescribers become familiar with one or two antidepressants from within each of the major classes, rather than spread experience thinly across many drugs.
- The newer antidepressants are considerably more expensive than the older ones. Yet although costs cannot be ignored, they are but a fraction of the overall cost of treating depressive disorder.
- Although meta-analyses suggest little difference in efficacy between older and newer antidepressants, an exception may be severe depression treated in hospital psychiatric units, for which the evidence from mixed-age studies favours tricyclics over SSRIs (BAP).

The main mode of action, the average starting dosages and therapeutic ranges of the most commonly prescribed antidepressants are shown in Box 8.6 (PTD, EXP). As regards mode of action (column 2), this is not an exact science as many antidepressants have dual action, affecting both noradrenaline (norepinrephine) and serotonin.

Box 8.6 Side-effect profiles and dosages of the main antidepressants (PTD, EXP)

Drug	*Main mode of action*	*Anticholinergic*	*Antihistaminic*	*α_1 Adrenergic blocking*	*Starting dosage (mg)*	*Average daily dose (mg)*
Amitriptyline	NE++ 5HT+	++++	++++	++++	25–50	75–100*
Imipramine	NE++ 5HT+	+++	++	+++	25	75–100*
Nortriptyline	NE++ 5HT+	+++	++	++	10–30	40–100
Dothiepin (dosulepin)	NE++ 5HT+	+++	++	++	50–75	75–150*
Mianserin	α_2	0/+	+++	0/+	30	30–90
Lofepramine	NE++ 5HT+	+	+	+	70–140	70–210
Trazodone	$5HT_2$	0	+++	+	100	300
Fluvoxamine	5HT	0/+	0/+	0	25–50	100–200
Sertraline	5HT	0/+	0	0	25–50	50–100
Fluoxetine	5HT	0/+	0	0	10	20
Paroxetine	5HT	0/+	0	0	10–20	20–30

Citalopram	5HT	0/+	0	0	10–20	20–30
Phenelzine	Monoamine oxidase inhibition (non-reversible)	0/+	0	++	15	30–45 (divided doses)
Moclobemide	RIMA	0/+	0	0	300	300–450
Venlafaxine XR	NE+ 5HT++	0/+	0	0/+	25–75	75–200
Mirtazepine	α_2 $5HT_2$	0	++	0	7.5–15	15–30
Bupropion SR	NE++/DA+	0/+	+	0	100	150–300
Nefazodone	$5HT_2$	0	+	+	50–100	150–300

5HT = serotonin reuptake inhibitor; NE = norepinrephine (noradrenaline) reuptake inhibitor; DA = dopamine reuptake inhibition; α_2 = antagonism at the presynaptic α_2 receptor. α_2+/++ indicates magnitude of effect from small (+) to marked (++++). *Titrate cautiously

Speed of onset

Research has consistently shown that, compared to younger adults, elderly people take longer to recover from a depressive episode (NIH). However, studies have not shown important differences between antidepressant drugs as regards speed of onset. However, if a dose titration interval is required, as with the older tricyclics, this will add to the time taken to recovery.

Because older patients take longer to recover than younger ones, a therapeutic trial in an older person may last up to 12 weeks. This is discussed further below.

Type of depression

Psychotic (delusional depression) A number of studies have indicated that in this subtype either a combination of an antidepressant used in conjunction with an antipsychotic drug (major tranquilliser) or ECT is more effective than an antidepressant given alone. In one recent study the combination of the tranquilliser perphenazine with an antidepressant was no more effective than an antidepressant alone (Mulsant et al, 2001). However, perphenazine is a relatively low-potency neuroleptic. The US Expert Panel (EXP) recommends combining an antidepressant with an antipsychotic. It provides guidelines for the use of antipsychotics (although generally this will be under specialist supervision):

- Haloperidol: starting does 0.5 mg; target dose 0.5–5 mg
- Olanzapine: starting does 2.5 mg; target dose 2.5–10 mg
- Perphenazine: starting dose 2–4 mg; target range 4–20 mg
- Quetiapine: starting dose 25–50 mg; target range 50–300 mg
- Risperidone: starting dose 0.25–0.5 mg; target range 0.5–4 mg.

Efficacy in special patient groups

Dementia

There is a high rate of placebo response in studies of antidepressants given to patients with dementia. With this in mind, for those with mild symptoms it is best to offer support to the patient and caregiver and review the situation over the next 4 weeks (the time within which most placebo responders have occurred in therapeutic trials).

If treatment is indicated because of intensity or duration of symptoms, then the following drugs have all been reported as being superior to placebo:

- Moclobemide in dosages of between 50 and 450 mg (Roth et al, 1996).
- Citalopram (Nyth et al, 1992).
- Sertraline and venlafaxine XR (EXP).

It is recommended that antidepressants be given with supportive psychotherapy to the patient along with focused caregiver support (EXP). There is some evidence (WPA) that SSRIs are effective in reducing symptoms in dementia such as agitation and food refusal, which may have their basis in affective disorder. In some studies improvement in cognition has been observed after depression in dementia has been treated (WPA).

Medical illness

Importantly, in a Cochrane meta-analysis (Gill & Hatcher, 1999) antidepressants used in a range of physical disorders were associated with an NNT of four, the same as the meta-analysis of Wilson et al (2001). As comorbidity is the rule in treating later-life depression this is an encouraging finding, although the analysis was not specific to older people.

If depressive symptoms are due to an underlying physical disorder, for example hypothyroidism, it is recommended that treatment for both conditions be initiated simultaneously (EXP). If they are due to a prescribed medication, then the choice is either to swap the medication or to continue it but coprescribe an antidepressant, depending on the clinical situation (EXP). Lastly, if depression is secondary to substance misuse, then the recommendation is first to treat the substance misuse and only prescribe antidepressants if the depression persists (EXP).

As regard specific trials in older medically ill people, there have been successful ones using fluoxetine (Evans et al, 1997) and lofepramine (Tan et al, 1994). Two aspects of particular interest in these studies are: in the fluoxetine trial patients with the most grave physical illness responded as well or better than less physically ill patients; and in the lofepramine trial there was benefit even though the dosage was deliberately kept at 70 mg (lower than that recommended). There is uncertainty as to whether low-dose antidepressants have a place in the management of frail older people. There has been some evidence (Tan et al, 1994) but also persisting doubts (Wilson et al, 2001).

Cole et al (2000) calculated that between 38 and 87% of elderly medically ill inpatients have contraindications to the use of older heterocyclic antidepressants, but only 4% to SSRIs (Cole et al, 2000). Not surprisingly, then, the drugs recommended for treating depression with physical comorbidity are SSRIs, bupropion, venlafaxine, mirtazepine and nefazodone, with SSRIs being the top choice (EXP). An exception is chronic non-malignant pain, where low dose tricyclics still have the advantage (EXP).

Stroke

In a review of antidepressants in stroke, Gustafson et al (1995) do not recommend the use of the older tricyclic antidepressants because of the high rate of contraindications and side effects, including delirium. As with dementia, there is a high rate of spontaneous recovery, but this diminishes rapidly after 6 weeks (Andersen et al, 1994). The following antidepressants have been shown to be superior to placebo in stroke: citalopram (Andersen et al, 1994) and fluoxetine (Wiart et al, 2000).

Nursing-home residents

Few studies have been conducted on this population. This is an important gap in knowledge, as these patients are likely to encompass the most difficult to treat, namely the very old and the very frail.

Tricyclic antidepressants have been shown to be effective but associated with unacceptably low tolerability (WPA). In an open study of SSRIs (Trappler & Cohen, 1998) the response rate was poor if the patient had associated dementia, but otherwise good. Likewise, in an open pilot study with sertraline in patients with minor (subthreshold) depression, outcome and tolerability were good (Rosen et al, 2000).

At present the best advice that can be offered is to treat cautiously with an SSRI or moclobemide, starting with a low dose and titrating upwards. An alternative is to deploy psychosocial interventions – in one study a socialisation programme was associated with short-term benefit (Rosen et al, 1997).

Tolerability

All antidepressants have side effects. It has been argued that the more serious ones occur with the tricyclics (with the exception of lofepramine, which is much safer) and that data from mixed-age patients in therapeutic trials indicate slightly lower drop-out rates for the SSRIs (BAP). In theory, the increased vulnerability of older people to side effects should make the newer drugs such as the SSRIs even better tolerated among the elderly than in younger patients, but this has not been proved. In fact, if older frail people are less tolerant of SSRI side effects, then the opposite might be true.

The more dangerous side effects, such as those affecting cardiac function and blood pressure, arise from treatment with the older drugs. The newer ones have a more benign profile. However, it is how the patient feels that matters. It is not only dangerous side effects that cause patients to discontinue treatment. In practice, even under rigorously controlled conditions 20% and 30% of patients drop out of antidepressant trials (WPA).

In terms of treatment-related effects, there is more evidence linking them to residual depressive symptoms than there is to the side effect of antidepressants, certainly for nortriptyline in the elderly (Marraccini et al, 1999).

The main side effects caused by anticholinergic, antihistaminic and adrenergic blockade are listed in Box 8.7 and by severity in Box 8.6. For the SSRIs, the major side effects are listed in Box 8.8.

The following additional points are important:

- Prior to commencing a tricyclic antidepressant, lying and standing blood pressure should be checked. A drop of 20 mmHg or more is likely to be aggravated by this class of drugs and lead to symptoms or falls. Postural hypotension is more likely in patients taking diuretic drugs or with poor left ventricular function (PTD).

Box 8.7 Side effects of tricyclics

Anticholinergic	*Antihistaminic*	*Adrenergic* (α_1 blockade)
Dry mouth	Oversedation	Postural hypotension
Blurred vision	Weight gain	
Constipation		
Urinary retention		
Cardiotoxicity		
Delirium		

Box 8.8 Side effects of SSRIs

- Nausea (around 15%)
- Diarrhoea (around 10%)
- Insomnia (5–15%)
- Anxiety/agitation (2–15%)
- Sexual dysfunction (up to 30% of younger people)
- Headache
- Weight loss
- Hyponatraemia/inappropriate antidiuretic hormone (ADH) secretion
- Discontinuation syndromes

- In some countries a baseline EKG (ECG) is recommended prior to commencement of tricyclic antidepressants.
- Tricyclic antidepressants have been given without adverse effects in patients with cardiac failure, provided it is stable (NIH).
- Tricyclic antidepressants can occasionally precipitate delirium to medically ill patients (PTD, WPA).

Because it is hardly ever enquired about, the occurrence of sexual dysfunction among older patients taking SSRIs is not known. By extrapolation from data on younger adults it is probably more common than thought.

Hyponatraemia, defined as a serum sodium of less than 135 mmol/ml, may be caused by an inappropriate secretion of antidiuretic hormone (ADH). It has been reported with all the SSRIs and venlafaxine but its true prevalence is unknown, as is its frequency complicating other classes of antidepressants (Kirby & Ames, 2001).

Discontinuation syndrome is characterised by rebound anxiety, insomnia, paraesthesiae and other symptoms, which can be confused with a relapse of depression. Although usually self-limiting, it may result in the patient losing confidence in the medication. Although reported most with paroxetine (and least with fluoxetine), discontinuation may occur as a result of abruptly stopping any antidepressant. Therefore antidepressants should always be tapered off, over a recommended period of 4 weeks (BAP).

If a change from one antidepressant to another is indicated it is not necessary to completely stop one drug before commencing the next, with the exception of moclobemide, for which there are special circumstances – the local formulary should be consulted.

An example of a cross-tapering regimen is as follows: changing from dothiepin 150 mg to citalopram 20 mg:

- Dothiepin: week 1 = 100 mg; week 2 = 50 mg; week 3 = 25 mg; week 4 = 0 mg
- Citalopram: weeks 1&2 = 10 mg; weeks 3&4 = 20 mg.

Note that fluoxetine can be stopped more quickly but can interact with tricyclics for several weeks after it has been stopped.

Safety

The newer antidepressants are much safer in overdose than the traditional tricyclics. Choosing a newer antidepressant may well be prudent if self-harm is a concern, but most overdoses in older people are not of antidepressants but analgesics (PTD, WPA). In other words, choosing a safer antidepressant is just one component of managing suicide risk.

Drug interactions
Some of the SSRIs interfere with liver cytochrome mechanisms, causing potential problems with drugs such as warfarin. Data sheets should be consulted.

Adjunctive medication (Box 8.9)
For patients disturbed by pervasive anxiety symptoms or insomnia the choice lies in either prescribing a drug with sedative effects, such as an older tricyclic or mirtazepine (for insomnia), or co-prescribing a short-acting benzodiazepine or hypnotic, respectively. Long-acting benzodiazepines are to be avoided (EXP). Another strategy is to coprescribe a course of trazodone, a mild antidepressant (EXP).

Box 8.10 provides a summary of those factors which are most important in selecting an antidepressant and those which are less so.

Newer themes and issues for future research

From the discussion it will be apparent that each class of antidepressant has its advantages and disadvantages. In many countries over recent years there has been a shift away from older tricyclic antidepressants to SSRIs. For example, in the PROSPECT study described earlier, the SSRI citalopram is recommended as first-line treatment. The WPA review suggests that citalopram and sertraline are the two SSRIs with the least propensity for interaction with other drugs. However, other experts have eschewed the notion of 'first-line treatment' as too simplistic (Roose & Suthers, 1998), although long-term studies are beginning to show that tricyclics are associated with reduced scores on health-related quality of

Box 8.9 Adjunctive medication

- Delusional depression – antipsychotic (or ECT)
- Anxiolytics, short-term, short half-life (e.g. lorazepam)
- Hypnotic, short-term (e.g. zopiclone) or trazodone

Box 8.10 Considerations in selecting an antidepressant

Factors that matter

- Age-associated pharmacokinetics (less important for newer antidepressants) (Ia)
- Depression type (e.g. psychotic/non-psychotic) (Ib)
- Prior response to a particular agent (III)
- Tolerability (Ib)
- Safety (Ia)
- Potential side effects (Ia)
- Drug interactions (Ia)
- Likely compliance (IIa)
- Comorbidity (dementia, physical disorder) (IIa)

Factors that are less important

- Efficacy (all are about equally effective) (Ib)
- Speed of action (all are about the same) (Ib)

Summary of evidence in relation to antidepressant drugs in the acute phase of treatment

- They are effective in older patients with a moderate to severe depressive episode (Ia)
- There are no important differences in speed of onset, although in general older people take longer to recover than younger adults (Ia–IIb)
- Their efficacy in acute minor (subthreshold) depression and uncomplicated grief is unproven (Ib)
- There is some evidence, although not extensive, that antidepressants may be effective in dysthymia in older people (Ib)
- Antidepressants are effective in patients with a range of physical comorbid conditions, but tolerability varies (Ia)
- Antidepressants are effective in the treatment of depression associated with dementia (Ib)

Recommendations for practice – acute treatment phase with antidepressants

- Patients with a moderate to severe depressive episode can be successfully treated with an antidepressant drug (A)
- For persistent minor depression (>4 weeks) an antidepressant trial should be considered (B)
- In primary care SSRIs are favoured as the first line of treatment in many countries (D)
- Patients with severe depressive episode being treated in psychiatric units should be considered for tricyclic antidepressant treatment (B)
- Older antidepressants should be avoided in patients at risk of suicide (D)
- If an older tricyclic is to be prescribed it is recommended that blood pressure (including postural drop) and EKG (ECG) be checked (D)
- For patients with moderate to severe depression in dementia treatment with an SSRI, moclobemide or venlafaxine is recommended, along with support to the caregiver (B)
- It is recommended that post-stroke depression be treated with an SSRI (C)
- In patients with comorbidity the recommended antidepressants are SSRIs, bupropion SR, venlafaxine, mirtazepine and nefazodone (D)
- There is insufficient evidence to recommend low-dosage antidepressants in major depression (B)
- In frail patients it is advisable to 'start low, go slow' (D)
- Given the range of antidepressants available, it may be advisable to become familiar with one or two agents from the main classes (D)

life measures, and perhaps deleterious effects on the cardiovascular system, such as a persistent mild elevation in the resting heart rate (Roose & Suthers, 1998). What is also clear is that there is a paucity of efficacy data concerning the oldest-old, especially regarding the newer antidepressants. Finally, the issue of whether low-dosage antidepressants are effective in older frail patients requires further research.

Patients who do not respond to first-line treatment in the acute phase

Knowing what to give the patient is only the first step. It is equally important to be knowledgeable about each step in the treatment. If at 4 weeks there has been little or no response to medication given in adequate dosage to a patient who is compliant, then recovery is unlikely (PTD, EXP). If the dosage is subtherapeutic it can be increased; otherwise, it is advisable to change to another antidepressant, preferably from another class. However, if recovery is under way – and this can be verified clinically by a rule of thumb of approximately one-quarter improvement on a rating scale such as the Hamilton Depression Rating scale or the Montgomery–Asberg (see Appendix) – then treatment can be continued (PTD, EXP) but the dosage may need to be optimised. If after a further 4 weeks the patient has improved but has not recovered then a further 4 weeks of treatment can be offered with the same antidepressant, but augmentation can also be considered at this point. Examples from the PROSPECT study (Mulsant et al, 2001) include buproprion SR 200–400 mg in two divided dosages; nortriptyline or lithium. Unless experienced with dual-drug regimens the practitioner should consider referral to a specialist. An alternative strategy is to switch to an antidepressant from another class. In the United States class switching is mainly from SSRIs to venlafaxine or bupropion (EXP). In the UK other options include lofepramine, which is not available in the United States.

Clearly these guidelines should not be interpreted too rigidly. For example, in partially responsive patients there is no certainty as to whether it is best to augment with the same antidepressant or to switch to another class. There are advantages and disadvantages in each approach (Box 8.11). Also, if the patient is in distress, waiting may not be acceptable and a referral for more intensive treatment such as ECT may be warranted.

Lastly, emerging evidence suggests that combining an antidepressant with a psychological therapy, such as CBT, IPT, problem-solving or psychodynamic psychotherapy, leads to a more favourable outcome than either treatment alone (EXP).

Electroconvulsive therapy (ECT)

Electroconvulsive therapy (ECT) has often been criticised and frequently ill-understood. Of all treatments available for moderate to severe depressive disorder it is the most effective (at about 80% recovery rate), and this is as true of older patients as younger ones. In fact, compared to younger patients, there is evidence that it is more effective. In one study it was almost a fifth more effective, and the benefits were manifest even among the oldest-old (Tew et al, 1999).

There is no consensus as to whether unilateral or bilateral ECT is the optimum method for older patients, although fixed-dose scheduling

Box 8.11 Factors favouring augmentation or substitution regimens (after Mulsant et al, 2001)

Augmentation	*Substitution*
Maintains improvement already achieved in partial responders	Avoids potential drug–drug interactions
Prevents delays associated with withdrawal of existing drug	Simpler regimen
Synergistic effects on two neurotransmitter systems	Lower costs
Allows current partially successful agent to be continued for longer	Easier to attribute side effects and understand tolerance

Summary of evidence for potential strategies in the patient who does not respond to first-line treatment (PTD, BAP)

- Extending the length of trial in partial responders may result in improvement in up to 50% more patients (IIa)
- Switching class from one antidepressant to another is associated with response rates of 50% in uncontrolled series, and lower rates in prospective trial data on younger patients (IIb)
- Augmentation with lithium salts may be effective in about 50% of patients – with retrospective studies reporting higher rates than prospective ones – but toxicity may occur in 11–23%. Regular blood monitoring is required for lithium (IIb)
- In mixed-age patients with more rigorously defined resistant depression both venlafaxine and ECT have been reported to show rates of recovery in between 30 and 50%, respectively (IIb)
- Within the emerging concept of vascular depression there is some evidence of a lower response to antidepressant monotherapy, but the response rate to ECT may be as favourable as for other patients, albeit with an increased risk of ECT-induced delirium (III)

Recommendations for practice – the poorly responsive patient (PTD). Strength of recommendation C

- If little or no response (<25% change in symptoms) by 4 weeks
  - Increase the dose, *or*, if dosage optimal
  - Change to another antidepressant (substitution)
- If partial response (25–50% improvement in symptoms) by 4 weeks:
  - Increase dose (if not already optimal)
  - Continue for further 2–4 weeks
  - Consider augmentation (see text)

- If little further improvement:
  - Augment, *or*
  - Substitute another class
- At any stage ECT may be the preferred option
- Psychological treatment may be used adjunctively with some evidence of improved outcome

may be more effective than dose titration (WPA). Bilateral ECT has been associated with greater efficacy and shorter treatment trials, but unilateral ECT with fewer adverse effects on memory.

ECT is highly effective in psychotic (delusional) depressive disorder and is often considered as the treatment of first choice for it (PTD, WPA), and it can be life-saving in patients who refuse to eat or drink adequately or who are actively suicidal (NIH). Symptoms that predict a positive response to ECT are similar at all ages, generally favouring patients with melancholic symptomatology (guilt, agitation, marked loss of interest, worthlessness and delusions), but in addition older depressed patients with marked anxiety respond too (PTD, WPA). Patients with dementia and depression can be given ECT with good effect, but post-ECT delirium is a greater risk (Rao & Lyketsos, 2000; PTD, WPA).

Although ECT is unlikely to be utilised by non-specialists, it is important to have sufficient knowledge so that referral is not delayed. There are no absolute contraindications to the administration of ECT (PTD) (Box 8.12).

Although the benefits of ECT are not reduced in older patients, those who are selected for this mode of treatment may constitute a subgroup with a high risk of later dementia (Brodaty et al, 2000). ECT can be given safely to patients with dementia and is effective, albeit with a high rate of transient delirium (Rao & Lyketsos, 2000).

Box 8.12 ECT – indications (EXP)

- Patient actively suicidal
- Urgent treatment to prevent deterioration in health (including food/fluid refusal)
- Psychotic depression
- Inadequate response to two trials of medication
- Intolerance to medication
- Prior good response

Psychological treatments

We have devoted considerable space to antidepressant treatment because that is where most evidence of efficacy lies. However, there is also good evidence of the effectiveness of psychological interventions; indeed, new evidence is emerging all the time. There is a general view, said to have originated from Freud himself (but in fact later retracted), that older people are not responsive to psychological therapies. This is incorrect: age is not a barrier to psychological intervention. Unfortunately, there is evidence that the legacy of the Freudian fallacy lives on. In a study of over 700 family physicians in the United States, although most thought that antidepressants were effective in older people, many were less optimistic about the effectiveness of psychotherapy (Gallo et al, 1999).

Three meta-analyses (Cuijpers 1998; Gatz et al, 1998; Pinquart & Sorensen, 2001) have provided evidence of efficacy in depression for the following interventions:

- Cognitive behaviour therapy (CBT) and behaviour therapy
- Interpersonal therapy (IPT)
- Brief psychodynamic psychotherapy
- Problem-solving therapy
- Life review for individuals with depressive symptoms or living in situations with restricted independence.

One study has shown an advantage for rational treatments, such as CBT, over emotive ones such as dynamic psychotherapy, but the difference was small (McCusker et al, 1998). CBT is an effective treatment on its own in moderate major depressive disorder (Thompson et al, 2001b). In a sample of medically ill patients with minor depression (Mossey et al, 1996), a course of six to eight sessions of interpersonal counselling given to 76 patients was more effective at 6, but not at 3, months than usual care.

Problem-solving treatment, of proven efficacy in younger patients with mild to moderate depression, has some evidence in favour of it in older subjects (Arean et al, 1993). It is based on CBT principles but, unlike CBT, requires only a moderate amount of training and can be taught to non-psychiatrically trained health professionals. As such, it offers promise in the treatment of older people with depressive episodes, especially in primary care. However, in a carefully designed study of older patients in primary care (Williams et al, 2000) it was no more effective than placebo plus clinical management, and less effective than paroxetine for both minor depression and dysthymia. A difficulty highlighted in this study was the enormous variation in efficacy across participating sites, with the more effective sites deploying more experienced therapists. Therefore, until problem-solving therapy can be standardised it cannot be recommended for milder (minor) depressive disorders.

Of those studies comparing antidepressants with psychotherapies and with combined treatments, the latter appear to be more effective in severe major depression than either given alone. Importantly, this appears to be true even if there has been a clear trigger for depression, such as bereavement (Reynolds et al, 1999b).

In the meta-analysis of McCusker et al (1998) non-specific interventions were also associated with improvement in depression, so it is important not to dismiss the inexpensive 'technologies' such as simple support. Likewise, a structured family intervention to those caring for a person with dementia, delivered along CBT principles, is associated with significant improvement in distress and depressive symptomatology (Marriot et al, 2000).

Summary of evidence – Psychotherapy

- The strongest evidence of efficacy exists for CBT and IPT (Ib)
- There is some evidence too of efficacy for brief dynamic psychotherapy, problem-solving therapy and life review (Ib–IIa)
- Psychotherapy is effective as a main treatment for older patients with moderate major depressive episodes (Ib)
- It is effective when combined with medication in severe major depression, and the combination is more effective than either modality alone (Ib)
- Problem-solving therapy may be an effective treatment for subthreshold (minor) depression, but only when the personnel delivering it have been trained to a consistent level (Ib)
- Offering support to patients and their caregivers is not the same as doing nothing. Simple support is associated with fairly high rates of symptom resolution in mild depression (Ib).
- A structured family intervention to caregivers of people with dementia has been shown to reduce depressive symptoms (Ib)

Recommendations for practice – psychotherapy

- It is recommended that primary care teams treating elderly depressed patients have access to personnel with training in either CBT or IPT (A)
- Wherever possible, supportive care should be offered to the patient and, where relevant, the caregiver (B)
- It is recommended that psychological interventions be available to patients with mild-to-moderate major depression as a first choice treatment (A)

Newer themes and areas for future research

The question of whether CBT techniques should be modified for use with older people is open to question. In a recent review it was concluded that CBT may be just as effective in older people without major modification (Laidlaw, 2001). Lastly, it is hoped that future research will clarify the role of problem-solving therapy, a relatively inexpensive psychological treatment.

Other treatment modalities

Between 1975 and 1990 Scogin and McElreath (1994) undertook meta-analyses of studies of psychosocial interventions in older depressed patients. This included broad-based approaches (for example self-help manuals) as well as formal psychotherapies. There was clear evidence in favour of active intervention. In a study of regular socialisation introduced into a long-term care facility, efficacy was apparent, although only for a maximum of 2 months after the intervention ended (Rosen et al, 1997). Family therapy has been adapted for use with older clients, and there are case reports of its efficacy in both dementia and depression (PTD, WPA).

The effects of exercise on mood are as yet not clear, although there are some associations. For example, in a large community sample increased rates of exercise were associated with fewer depressive symptoms, but there was no effect of exercise on incident depression (Kritz-Silverstein et al, 2001) or only a very modest effect (Morgan & Bath, 1998), whereas in a Finnish study (Lampinen et al, 2000) decreasing exercise was associated with an increased risk of depression.

Music therapy is sometimes used in older patients, and there is modest evidence of its efficacy in depression (WPA).

Collaborative care

Managing depressive disorder in an older person is not simply a matter of selecting the right intervention from a range of medications and psychological therapies. Holistic care is important. Improvements in factors such as medical care, attempting to engender a positive adaptive style of coping and good social support may aid recovery from depression (PTD). Input may be needed from a range of practitioners – social worker, psychologist, occupational therapist, podiatrist, dietitian and physiotherapist. A consensus is emerging that depressive disorder should be viewed in the same light as other chronic conditions and care delivered accordingly (von Korff & Goldberg, 2001). This will require a shift in resources and more collaboration between primary and secondary care.

Strategies in mixed-age studies which have *not* been shown to be effective include passive feedback of screening results to primary care physicians and dissemination of practice guidelines without a change in practice (Peveler & Kendrick, 2001). Data on older depressed subjects are limited, but also suggest that educational packages offered by a nurse to primary care physicians, feedback of screening test results, or simply recommending that antidepressants are prescribed to patients screened positive are insufficient to influence practice in primary (Livingston et al, 2000; Stevens et al, 1999; Whooley et al, 2000) or secondary care (Weatherall, 2000; Yohannes et al, 2000). However, a suitably trained nurse ('advanced practice nurse') who coordinates care is associated with improved outcomes in both primary care (McCurren et al, 1999; Rabins et al, 2000) and in hospital liaison (Kurlowicz, 2001). These data do not mean that education or screening are of no value, but that on current evidence they are unlikely to be effective as standalone strategies.

From studies of younger patients (Peveler & Kendrick, 2001; von Korff & Goldberg, 2001), strategies which have been associated with improved outcomes include the identification of a case manager (for example a practice nurse) who takes responsibility for following up patients, seeing that they adhere to their treatment plan and that it is adjusted when it is not working. Another facet of successful strategies involves integrating primary care services with those of specialist mental health services.

Some other elements of these models of care have involved telephone support (a relatively low-cost intervention) and improved access to psychiatrists (von Korff & Goldberg, 2001).

As regard older people, two studies have reported positive data on outcome for patients residing in the community. A community psychiatric nurse (CPN) from a specialist mental health team was more effective in the primary care management of depression in older people than usual treatment (Waterreus et al, 1994). This study compared a care management plan delivered by a CPN with GP controls. Compliance with medication was improved in this study. A research psychiatrist implementing a management plan in frail older depressed patients (defined by the amount of home care they received) was more effective than GP treatment alone (Banerjee et al, 1996) but this would be an expensive intervention.

Three studies have reported on the benefits of a collaborative approach in residential and nursing homes. A randomised controlled trial has examined the efficacy of a multifaceted intervention for residents of nursing homes who are depressed (Llewellyn-Jones et al, 1999). A model of care between the psychiatric team and primary care was developed, with interventions aimed at (a) increasing the detection rate of depression by carers; (b) encouraging older people to accept that depression is treatable; and (c) providing accessible treatment programmes in residential care. There were clinically important benefits. Primary care physicians remained in control of antidepressant medication, but there was regular contact between them and the specialist mental health team. The interventions included education to both the physicians and the residential care workers.

In another trial, over 100 residents of nursing and residential homes were randomly allocated to either usual care or an intervention from a nurse with psychiatric training, delivered along the lines of goal planning plus educational outreach visits by a local psychogeriatric outreach team. In unselected patients with either dementia or depression, there was improvement in cognition and depressed mood but not behavioural problems (Proctor et al, 1999). Lastly, a psychiatrically trained nurse working in conjunction with older adult volunteers, working as paraprofessionals, resulted in a reduction in depression scores (McCurren et al, 1999).

Summary of evidence – collaborative care

- Passive feedback of screening results, distributing guidelines and other educational material to primary care physicians are ineffective on their own (Ib)
- Shared care of depressive disorder has been shown to be effective in primary care and care homes for older and mixed-age patients (Ib)
- Compliance with medication improves with shared care for younger depressed patients (Ib), and there is some positive evidence too in older depressed patients (IIa)

Recommendations for practice (Category B)

There is insufficient evidence to recommend any one particular model, but the following are successful:

- Identifying a care coordinator (case manager),
- Active follow-up of patients,
- Giving educational packages to caregivers (in residential and nursing homes)
- Enhancing the links between primary and secondary care.

Resistant depression

There is no agreed definition of resistant depression. In fact, different levels of resistance to treatment can be set. One such system (Thase & Rush, 1997) is as follows:

- 0 No adequate trial of medication
- 1 Non-response to antidepressant monotherapy
- 2 Non-response to two trials of monotherapy from drugs of different classes
- 3 Stage 2 plus failure to respond to one augmentation strategy

- 4 Stage 3 plus failure of a second augmentation strategy
- 5 Stage 4 plus failure to respond to course of ECT.

As only 50–60% of patients are responsive to the first antidepressant they are prescribed, the primary care physician can expect to be involved in decision making at levels 1 and perhaps level 2 on a regular basis.

Experts on resistant depression frequently point out that many so-called resistant patients have never had even one adequate trial of an antidepressant (Bowskill & Bridges, 1997). It is therefore important to have a systematic approach to the management of patients not responding to first-line therapy. One such approach has been outlined (Guscott & Grof, 1991). The diagnosis may be incorrect: for example, a patient may be quietly harbouring psychotic ideation, which may not respond to an antidepressant on its own. The level of compliance may be low and there may be attendant health and/or psychosocial factors that impede recovery. For example, a patient may be investing in being an invalid in order to seek more attention from his or her family. If these factors have been addressed adequately, the physician is faced with making a decision to continue the medication, to augment it or to substitute it.

Guscott and Grof (1991) recommend using a stepped care approach in the management of depression. By this they mean that each intervention is planned in a logical way, one following on from another, rather than randomly. Although data are limited, there have been studies which have shown that if a stepped approach is utilised, the true prevalence of resistant depression in older patients drops to as low as 10%, at least in specialised settings (Flint & Rifat, 1995; Little et al, 1998).

New treatment modalities which may offer hope in resistant depressive disorder include transcranial magnetic stimulation (TMS) and vagal nerve stimulation. The latter is a specialist tool which has been used successfully in resistant depression in younger patients. TMS holds some promise as an alternative to other physical treatments such as ECT, but so far there is insufficient evidence to recommend its use in elderly patients.

Continuation therapy

This is the period after recovery during which treatment should be continued in order to lessen the chances of a relapse. Data are limited. Guidance for younger patients suggests a continuation period of 6 months for major depression. However, in the recent Expert Consensus (EXP) 56% of experts recommended treatment for 12 months in first-onset patients with major depression in later life, and two-thirds recommended treatment for 2 or more years in recurrent cases. In a study of preventative therapy with the antidepressant dothiepin (dosulepin) (Old Age Depression Interest Group, 1993) the majority of relapses occurred within the first 12 months of therapy, so that a minimum interval of 12 months seems justified. There are no data as regards non-major depression. Studies from primary care (for example Rojas-Fernandez et al, 1999) show that a substantial proportion of older people prescribed antidepressants are given them for an inappropriately short period of time. In the study cited half of prescriptions were for less than 6 months.

Maintenance therapy

There is evidence that over periods of up to 36 months, maintaining the patient on an antidepressant or giving IPT is superior to placebo in preventing recurrences of depression (Old Age Depression Interest Group, 1993; Reynolds III et al, 1999a; Bump et al, 2001). Antidepressants which have been shown to be effective in this way in older patients are the tricyclics dothiepin (dosulepin) and nortriptyline, and the SSRIs citalopram and paroxetine.

There are two views on maintenance therapy. One (Old Age Depression Interest Group, 1993) suggests that the avoidance of even a single episode in an older patient is a worthwhile aim, given that the older person may have only a few years of life ahead. The other (Roose & Suthers, 1998) argues that it is unwarranted to subject all older people with a history of depression to lifelong treatment with tablets which may have undesirable side effects with time. A compromise position, not backed by evidence, is to treat the patient for 12 months beyond recovery and then to discuss with the patient and his or her caregivers whether there are risk factors for recurrence in which case long-term treatment may be discussed. Lastly, maintaining the patient on the full dose of antidepressant rather than reducing it results in better protection against recurrence (NIH).

Summary of evidence – continuation and maintenance treatment

- Current evidence suggests a continuation period for a major depressive episode of 12 months for a first episode; longer for a recurrent disorder (Ib)
- There is little available evidence regarding non-major depression
- Effective maintenance for the prevention of recurrence has been demonstrated for nortriptyline, dosulepin, citalopram and paroxetine (Ib)
- There is a lack of consensus on how long maintenance treatment should last, or whether it should last for life (IV)

Recommendations for practice

- On current evidence patients with a first-onset major depression should be continued on the same dosage of antidepressant that improved them for 12 months (B)
- Those with recurrent depression should be continued at the same dosage that improved them, with a review at 12 months to discuss risk factors (C)
- For high-risk patients treatment should be continued for at least 3 years or indefinitely (C)

When to refer for specialist advice

Following the guidelines above, most patients will recover. However, some will not, and it is important to know which patients to refer for specialist advice. Delay has its cost, as persistence of symptoms in the acute phase of treatment increases the chances of chronic depression in the longer term. Box 8.13 summarises the chief reasons for referral to a specialist (PTD).

Box 8.13 When to refer (PTD, EXP)

- When the diagnosis is in doubt
- When depression is severe, as evidenced by:
  - Psychotic depression
  - Severe risk to health because of failure to eat or drink
  - Suicide risk
- Complex therapy is indicated (for example in cases with medical comorbidity)
- When first-line therapy fails (although more experienced physicians may wish to pursue a second course of a different antidepressant)

chapter 9

Course and outcome

Traditional teaching held the prognosis of depressive disorder to be benign. That it is a serious disorder with far-reaching consequences is not at odds with this, nor should it be regarded as a counsel of despair. Even when appropriately managed, not all recurrences can be prevented, although recurrent episodes do respond to effective management (NIH). A number of studies have clarified the long-term outlook for older patients. A meta-analysis by Cole and Bellavance (1997a), for hospital-based studies, which until recently were the most commonly reported, showed the following:

- Whether in the short term (24 months or less) or the longer term (more than 24 months), about 60% of patients with major depression either remained well, or had further relapses and/or recurrences which were treatable.
- Between 15 and 20% of patients can be expected to develop chronic depressive symptomatology. Although this is cause for concern, the majority of patients either stayed well or developed a relapse or recurrence which could be treated successfully.

Cole and Bellavance (1997a) attempted another analysis of older patients in the community. Only five studies could be found, so that detailed breakdown became imprecise. However, the findings were less favourable, with fewer than one-third having a good outcome. The reasons for this are unclear, but the authors reported antidepressant rates of only 4%, 9% and 33% in three of the community studies they cited. It seems more likely than not that the poor prognosis in community samples is related to low rates of treatment.

Lastly, Cole and Bellavance, in a further meta-analysis (Cole & Bellavance, 1997b), reported that only a fifth or less older patients with depression on medical wards were well at 3 months. Numbers were small but, given that depressive disorder is treatable in patients with medical illness, this is an alarming finding. Again, lack of appropriate treatment may be a factor.

Comparative outcomes

A common misconception is that late-life depression has a worse outcome than at other times of life. There have been a number of studies, six of which were reported by PTD, all showing outcomes in the elderly as good as or better than for younger depressed patients. Two recent studies have shown the opposite. In one (Tuma, 2000), recovery rates among adults aged under 65 were almost double those of the older comparison group, but the difference was largely accounted for by an increase in the development of dementia (15%) and of death (33%) in the older group. In the other, a large unblinded study of office-treated patients, chronicity was 13% more frequent in older than younger patients (Benazzi, 2000). The NIH panel report that the long-term outcome is broadly similar in younger and older patients, but with older patients being somewhat more susceptible to relapse. There are no comparison data for younger versus older primary care-treated patients. Negative expectations about the prospects for recovery from depression in older people is one probable reason for its undertreatment.

Non-suicide mortality

Data from several hospital-based series and of untreated community samples demonstrate a high rate of death among older people with major depression compared to age-matched controls. For example, in the study by Tuma (2000), over the period of study an expected rate of death would be about 5% year-on-year, giving an expected figure of about 22.5% as against the actual one of 33%. In other studies the reported rates are up to 2.5 times that expected. Other research has demonstrated that this excess cannot be entirely explained by the coexistence of poor health (PTD).

O'Brien and Ames (1994) postulate several possible mechanisms for the increased mortality in depression: comorbid physical illness; occult illness; illness effects (e.g. related to psychomotor retardation); treatment effects; biological effects such as abnormality of the hypothalamopituitary–adrenal-axis, or endocrine abnormalities. Immune dysfunction is a further possibility (Dentino et al, 1999). Undertreatment is another explanation. For example, in an older study cardiovascular mortality was found to be higher in elderly depressed men whose depression was judged to be inadequately treated (Avery & Winokur, 1976).

Prognostic factors

Comparatively little is known about which factors are important in outcome. Poorer outcomes may be linked to delays in initiating treatment and/or resolving symptoms. There is emerging evidence of a poorer outcome in patients with psychotic (delusional) depression and in patients with severe deep white matter abnormality as visualised on magnetic resonance imaging (MRI) (O'Brien et al, 1998).

The question of whether cognitive impairment and dementia are risk factors for a poorer outcome is of practical importance. Many of the studies cited above excluded patients with cognitive dysfunction. However, a number of studies of patients with measurable dysfunction at the index episode of depression have demonstrated high levels of later dementia even when the signs of cognitive impairment resolved with treatment of depression. In the past, some of these patients would have been termed 'pseudodemented', a term which we have avoided as it has no agreed clinical meaning. However, in practice it would seem prudent to follow up and observe for signs of dementia in those patients who present with depression and impaired cognition (evidenced by, say, poor performance on the Mini-Mental Status Examination).

One potentially important factor which is inconsistently linked to outcome is age at onset of depression. Some studies have shown a more favourable prognosis in early-onset depression, but others have shown the opposite (WPA).

More general factors which are associated with a poorer outcome represent adversity, hardship and poor health, some of which can and some cannot be modified. Emerging evidence comes from the finding that a

Summary of evidence – outcome factors

- The outcome of depressive disorder in older people is as good as in other age groups (Ia)
- There may be more susceptability to relapse (more 'brittle' outcomes) in older patients, although relapses can respond to treatment (Ib)
- The risk of relapse and recurrence can be reduced by antidepressant medication or IPT, or a combination of both (Ib)
- The prognosis in patients in the community and in medical wards is much worse, and the reasons for this are unclear (Ia)
- Prognostic factors may be divided into clinical features and more general factors (III):
  - *Clinical features:* slower initial recovery; more severe initial depression; duration >2 years; three or more previous episodes (for recurrence); previous history of dysthymia; psychotic symptoms; marked initial anxiety; extensive deep white matter and basal ganglia gray matter brain disease; cognitive impairment
  - *General factors:* chronic stress associated with poor environment, crime and poverty; a new physical illness or worsening of a physical illness; becoming a victim of crime; poor perceived (but not necessarily tangible) social support.

poor subjective perception of wellbeing is linked to recovery, so that taking account of how the patient views himself or herself is important. Depression also leads to reduced subjective feelings of wellbeing and poorer perceived health, so that the concepts are intimately linked. There is evidence that patients with poorer self-perceived health at baseline tend to comply less well with medical treatment, which is one explanation for their poor outcome (Lenze et al, 2001a).

On a more positive note, there is good evidence that maintenance antidepressant therapy, and/or adjunctive psychotherapy, is associated with low rates of recurrence (less than a third) over intervals up to 4 years (Taylor et al, 1999; Reynolds et al 1999a; Flint & Rifat, 2000).

Recommendations for practice – outcome

- It is recommended that major depression in older people be treated like other chronic disabling conditions, with attention to follow-up after recovery in the acute phase (C)
- It is recommended that patients who present with cognitive impairment when depressed (e.g. MMSE score below 24) be followed up for later signs of dementia (C)

Suicide

Recent data show that in 1999, in the United States 32 000 people killed themselves, 6200 of them elderly (Salvatore, 2000). From 1980 to 1992 the suicide rate among people aged over 65 in the United States rose by 9%. Most striking was a 35% increase in rates for men and women aged 80–84 years (NIH). The suicide rate in the US is six times that of the general population in those aged over 85 (NIH). In most societies where this has been studied, older people are overrepresented. At least two-thirds of older people who kill themselves are suffering from depressive disorder (Barraclough, 1971; Cattell & Jolley, 1995; Harwood et al, 2001). They also suffer significantly more physical illness and greater functional limitation than control subjects (Conwell et al, 2000).

A majority will have consulted their primary care physician in the preceding month (Barraclough, 1971; Cattell & Jolley, 1995), although they may be less likely to report suicidal thoughts (Duberstein et al, 1999). Only a quarter are likely to have been in contact with specialist mental health services. There are fewer consistent data on possible links with other psychiatric disorders, such as alcohol abuse and dementia. Personality factors have received less attention, but disorders of personality are probably relatively uncommon among elderly suicide victims than among younger ones, although some lifelong personality traits may be overrepresented, such as anankastic characteristics (Harwood et al, 2001) and introversion.

Identifying high-risk patients within primary care would appear to offer the best chance of reducing death by suicide in older people. Depressive disorder is the main predisposing factor, notably with a clinical picture characterised by severe agitation, guilt, hopelessness, insomnia and marked somatic preoccupation. Other factors include being male, especially (in some studies) a white male (Brown et al, 2001) and of greater age (>80 years); chronic painful conditions, functional limitation and social isolation are all important (Conwell et al, 2000). Rather than poor social circumstances contributing to suicide, an alternative model might be that better social conditions reduce vulnerability to it.

Caine (2001) has outlined three broad approaches to suicide prevention in older people: health maintenance and promotion; treatment of depression in primary care and community settings; and screening for suicidal ideation coupled with direct preventative efforts. With regard to the latter two strategies, the evidence of effectiveness is inconsistent. The Gotland study (Rutz et al, 1989) is the only example in which an educational programme to improve primary care physicians' knowledge of depression and its treatment reduced suicide rates (in this case for women only). The improvement, however, lasted only for 3 years, suggesting that an ongoing programme is necessary. In the United Kingdom, the replacement of coal gas with non-noxious natural gas resulted in reduced suicide rates, mainly among older people, suggesting that removing a means may have an important beneficial effect. As an example of how this might be implemented in practice, in the United States a study showed that those primary care physicians who asked older depressed people about access to firearms were more likely to have had expertise in geriatric mental health and training in risk assessment (Kaplan et al, 1998).

Also in the United States a major initiative (PROSPECT) has been mentioned earlier which uses a 'guided management' intervention for depression, hopelessness and suicidal ideation within a collaborative care model. Its aim is to test collaborative models which may lead to the early detection and prevention of suicide in older people by the accurate detection and appropriate management of depressive disorder. Data are awaited but its aims have been described (Brown et al, 2001).

Clearly, appropriate detection and adequate management of depressive disorder, especially within primary care, remain a priority for suicide prevention in older people. However, a broad-based public health approach may be appropriate. Thus poor health, chronic pain, disablement and social isolation are the context for depression and suicide, just as poor diet, lack of exercise and smoking are for heart disease (Caine, 2001).

There are more subtle ways in which suicidal ideation can lead to death. For example, in one study depressive symptoms were associated with greater interest in physician-assisted suicide, euthanasia and treatment refusal in medically ill inpatients (Blank et al, 2001), and with a greater likelihood of refusing cardiopulmonary resuscitation (Lifton & Kett, 2000).

Newer themes and issues for future research

- There is increasing recognition that outcome in late-life depression should address more than symptom resolution. Suggestions have included functional recovery, service use and quality of life (WPA). Studies are now beginning to document improvement in quality of life which comes with treatment of depression (Shmuely et al, 2001).

- The premise that the most appropriate way to reduce suicide among older people is by addressing depressive disorder in primary care is an important conceptual development. Studies are under way to address this.

Summary of evidence – suicide

- It is hard to predict which patients may attempt suicide, but there is growing evidence that identifying and managing depressive disorder in primary care is the most effective way to reduce suicide in older people (IV)
- The risk of suicide in older people can be divided into general factors and clinical features (IIa):
  - *General factors:* greater age (>80); male gender; living alone; inadequate social support; significant loss; alcohol abuse (not specific to elderly); cultural acceptability (in some societies more acceptable than others)
  - *Psychiatric factors:* past attempt; marked psychomotor agitation; insomnia; severe guilt; hopelessness; persistent hypochondriasis; suicidal ideation

Recommendations for practice – suicide risk

Until more definitive evidence becomes available, it is recommended that the strategy most likely to affect suicide rates is the effective identification and management of depressive disorder in primary care (D)

chapter 10

Prevention

Primary prevention

Primary prevention involves measures such as public health education, support for the bereaved, and strategies aimed at reducing the stigma of depression. There are many examples of local initiatives. Examples in the UK include *Defeat Depression* and the campaign *Changing Minds*, both sponsored by the Royal College of Psychiatrists. There are also many examples of locally produced leaflets and information sources. For example, in the United States the American Association of Geriatric Psychiatrists has a well produced booklet entitled *Depression in Late Life: not a natural part of aging* (www.aagpgpa.org).

Secondary prevention

This is aimed at reducing the risk of a recurrence and/or relapse of depression. The evidence has already been described and the appropriate recommendations are listed in Boxes 10.1 and 10.2. In practical terms this will involve timely and optimum treatment in the acute phase, and appropriate continuation treatment and prophylaxis, either with antidepressant treatment, psychological therapy or lithium salts, for those identified at high risk of recurrence (NIH, PTD). Without planned aftercare relapses and recurrences often go undetected (Baldwin, 2000). In

Box 10.1 Recommendations for prevention of relapse (PTD, NIH, EXP)

- Treat acute phase to remission of *all* symptoms (not elderly-specific) (A)
- Continue antidepressants for at last 12 months (new case) or longer (recurrent case) (B)
- For major depressive disorder, where possible combine pharmacological treatment with psychological therapy (B)
- Follow up patients where possible (C)

Box 10.2 Recommendations for prevention of recurrence (PTD, NIH, EXP)

- Identify patients at high risk of recurrence and treat with medication (SSRI or tricyclic) and/or psychological treatment (A)
- Consider maintenance ECT for high-risk cases (C)
- Follow up patients systematically where possible (C)

specialist settings there is some evidence from small case series of the efficacy of maintenance ECT (Prudec et al, 1994; WPA).

Tertiary prevention

This is aimed at reducing the disability associated with the continuation of depressive disorder. This will include support for patients, optimising medical conditions and support to caregivers, including the opportunity for respite breaks if needed (PTD).

chapter 11

Executive summary

Depressive disorder is the most common mental health problem of older people. Recently it has become clear that it is associated with very serious morbidity and a high rate of mortality. It is therefore important for the affected individual that it be managed appropriately, and that it is also regarded as a serious public health issue in society. What makes depression in later life different is not so much different symptoms, although there is increasing evidence for some new subtypes such as minor depression and vascular depression, but comorbidity. This arises from psychiatric illness such as dementia and a range of medical illnesses which occur often in older people, as well as from prescribed medication. Most evidence for treatment exists for antidepressant drugs, and with many new ones to choose from it is almost always possible to find a suitable antidepressant for an older patient. But it is also clear that psychological interventions are effective, either as the sole treatment for moderate major depression or adjunctively in more severe cases, although regrettably they are often less available to older than to younger people. The principles of treatment are not altered in later life, but comorbidity and frailty affect how and what treatment is given. Holistic care is most likely to be effective when it is multimodal and multidisciplinary. There are interesting new concepts regarding collaboration between specialist and primary care, and these have important implications for the management of older depressed patients. The prognosis is as good as for younger adults but is more brittle, so that it is important to offer continuation therapy and follow up patients. Another priority is to reduce suicide in older people, and the most effective strategy is likely to be through better recognition and management of depression in primary care. Lastly, for quick reference, the summary boxes of evidence and the practice recommendations are reproduced on the following pages.

Signs and symptoms of depression

Summary of evidence

- In older people depressive disorder can be distinguished from normal ageing (IIa)
- Major depressive disorder in older people often manifests in the same way as in younger adults (IIa)
- There is little evidence of a specific sub-type of major depression in older people (IIa)
- But several factors modify its presentation (IIb). These include:
  - A reduced complaint of sadness
  - Hypochondriasis and somatic concern instead of sadness
  - Poor subjective memory or a dementia-like picture
  - Marked anxiety
  - Apathy and poor motivation

Recommendations for practice

- In order to detect major depression in older people, it is important that practitioners are trained to recognise the leading symptoms as outlined in major classificatory systems such as ICD10 and DSM IV (B)
- Equally it is important to be aware of symptoms which are often the clue to an underlying depression in an older person. The most important of these are:
  - a reduced complaint of sadness, even when appearing depressed to others

- excessive preoccupation with health and physical symptoms
- when the patient is distressed by poor memory rather than depression (B)

Disease burden

Summary of evidence

- As a cause of suffering, depressive disorder is one of the leading causes world-wide (IIa)
- It is often not recognized or is inadequately treated (IIa)
- As a result it increases morbidity from associated conditions, pushes up costs and hastens death (IIa)
- With appropriate treatment quality of life is improved for the older person (Ib)

Recommendations for practice

- The enormous negative impact of depressive disorder in older people should be acknowledged in government policy and health planning (B)
- Practitioners should regard depressive disorder in older people as a serious and potentially chronic condition – like other seriously disabling conditions (B)
- Practitioners should have a low threshold for its detection, as it is frequently overlooked (B)
- Practitioners should become familiar with its management as it is often not treated optimally (B)

Types of depression

Summary of evidence

- A high proportion of clinically important depression in older people is non-major or sub-threshold depression (IIa)
- For every case of major depression in later life there are between two and three non-major ones (minor or sub-threshold depression) (IIa)
- Terms such as minor depression and sub-threshold depression are increasingly used to refer to this type of depression, although it is likely to be a heterogeneous category (IIa).
- Such cases do not meet criteria for ICD or DSM major depression, although in reality they are clinically important (IIb)
- There is evidence that these non-major depressions (minor or sub-threshold depressions) are nevertheless a significant cause of suffering and morbidity (IIa)
- There is also evidence that major and 'minor' depressions are on a continuum rather than quite separate disorders (IIa – extrapolated from mixed-aged populations)
- Minor (sub-threshold) depression in older people is sometimes characterised by a distinct symptom profile which includes poor concentration and amotivation in association with poorer health (IIa)
- Dysthymia is probably more common among older people than realised and is a risk factor for major depression (IIb)
- Another subtype occurs in patients who have late onset depression with vascular disease and evidence on neuroimaging of subcortical white matter and gray matter changes, so-called 'vascular depression' (IIb)
- Bipolar disorder is uncommon in later life but associated with considerable morbidity (IIb)
- Organic causes of depressive episode occur more frequently in older than younger patients (III)

Recommendations for practice

- In older people major depression, non-major depression and dysthymia are all targets for clinical intervention (B)
- Practitioners should be aware that sub-threshold (minor) depression is a significant disorder and not a trivial one (B)
- It is important to have a high index of suspicion for sub-threshold (minor) depression, particularly in people with poor health who have low mood, impaired cognition and low motivation (B)
- In older depressed people it is important to rule out organic causes (C)

Prevalence

Summary of evidence

- Around one in every eight older people living in the community will have clinically important depressive symptoms, with women having higher rates then men (IIa)
- Although some societies report lower rates, the prevalence is remarkably consistent internationally (IIa)
- Among older people being attended by a primary care physician the prevalence is roughly doubled (IIa)
- Being in receipt of a high level of home support is associated with a rate of depression, about double that of less frail community-dwelling elders (IIa)
- Rates of depression are exceptionally high in hospitals and residential and nursing home facilities (IIa)

Recommendations for practice

- Depressive disorder, disability and dependency are all highly correlated. In general, the more disability the more depression. It is always worth considering depression in settings where disability is high, such as hospital wards, residential and nursing homes and the frail elderly at home (B)
- It is important to have a low threshold (high index of suspicion) for diagnosing depression in these settings and also among patients consulting in primary care (B)

Aetiology

Summary of evidence for causative factors in depression in later life

- **Predisposing factors**
  - Female gender (IIa)
  - A prior history of depressive disorder (IIa)
  - Widow/widowerhood; being divorced (IIa)
  - Alteration in brain neuroamines and receptors (evidence mixed; not conclusive)
  - Neuroendocrine disturbance (evidence mixed; not conclusive)
  - Brain changes – mild atrophy; white matter and other changes; reduced perfusion (III – associative findings; clear causal findings unproven)
  - Personality – reduced capacity to form abiding attachments (IIb)
  - Physical co-morbidity; disability & handicap (IIa)
  - Medication, alcohol and systemic disease (IIa)
  - Caregiving (IIa)
  - Social disadvantage (IIa)
  - Lack of social support (IIa)

- **Precipitating factors**
  - Adverse life events (IIa)
  - Chronic stress (IIb)
- **Protective factors**
  - Optimal medical care (III)
  - Positive coping style (III)
  - Social support (IIa)

Recommendations for practice

- In practice it is important to take a multi-factorial approach to causation in depression, recognising the roles of both individual susceptibility and adverse life events (B)
- Organic factors are often important in depressive disorder of older people; it is important to take a drug and alcohol history, including over-the-counter analgesics (B)
- Disability due to physical ill-health is strongly associated with depressive disorder; it should therefore be minimised as much as possible (B)
- Good medical care may reduce the incidence of depression or reduce its impact (C)
- The concept of handicap places disability in a social context. It is strongly associated with onset of depression and much handicap can be prevented (B)
- Positive social and environmental factors (including the level and quality of support) may offset some of the negative effects of adverse life events and are important areas for intervention (B/C)

Co-morbidity

Summary of evidence

- Depression in older people often co-exists with other psychiatric symptoms such as anxiety. (IIa)
- Dementia is associated with a high rate of co-morbid depression (IIa)
- Frailty, disability and dependency are highly correlated with depressive disorder in older people (Ib)
- Some physical disorders may predispose to or cause depression. Those most frequently encountered are stroke, Parkinson's disease, hip fracture, cancer, myocardial infarction, heart failure and chronic pulmonary disease (IIa)
- For stroke and heart disease and perhaps cancer and hip fracture there is evidence that depressive disorder itself predisposes to these conditions (IIa)
- In practice physicians tend to focus on either the physical or the mental and not both (IIb)
- Some physical disorders seem able to precipitate depression via a direct effect on the brain neurotransmitter systems such as serotonin (IIb)
- Other disorders exert an effect through a more complex interplay of physical, psychological and social factors (IIa)

Recommendations for practice

- In order to achieve optimal outcomes for the patient both mental and physical health problems should be treated together, as the prognosis of the one is closely associated with that of the other. (A)
- In dementia it is important to check for signs and symptoms of depression, as it is common (B)
- It is important to check for signs and symptoms of depression in patients with Parkinson's disease, heart disease, chronic

pulmonary disease or who have had a stroke or hip fracture as they are at high risk of depression (B).

- It is worth asking the patient about adverse life events prior to a serious medical illness, as it may have been involved in causing depression and it may require intervention in its own right (for example bereavement counselling) (C)

Screening

Summary of evidence – screening questionnaires for depressive disorder in older people (evidence level Ib–IIb)

- GDS (4, 5, 10 12, 15 and 30-item versions)
- Cornell Scale for depression in dementia
- BASDEC
- EASY-care

Recommendations for targeted screening in primary care (level B)

- Recent major physical illness (within 3 months)
- Chronic handicapping illness
- Receiving high level of home support (personal care)
- Recent bereavement (3–6 months)
- Socially isolated older people
- Those who persistently complain of loneliness
- Patients with persistent sleep difficulties

Assessment

Summary of evidence

- Clinical knowledge, appropriate attitudes to older people and good interview skills will lessen the chances of over looking depressive disorder (IV)
- A diagnosis of depressive disorder is the leading risk factor for suicide in older people. (IIa)
- A comprehensive assessment of depressive disorder in an older person includes taking a history, performing an assessment of the mental state and of risk, carrying out a relevant physical examination and requesting a range of appropriate tests (IV)
- The investigations most relevant are a blood count, serum chemistry, thyroid function, B_{12} and folate (IV)
- Those most at risk of suicide are isolated men aged over 80 with a previous history of attempting self harm; those who have chronic often painful conditions or who abuse alcohol or pills; or who have a clinical picture of severe depression (III)
- Most older people who have killed themselves have seen their primary care physician within the preceding month (IIa)
- There are number of reliable instruments which can be used to rate depressive symptoms (Ib).

Recommendations for practice

The recommendations constitute Category D evidence. This is an area where practice is informed as much by experience as research. Current best practice regarding assessment of the older person is that the following should be conducted on patients presenting with depressive disorder:

- History
- Mental state
- Risk assessment for suicide and non-deliberate self-harm

- Focused physical and neurological examination
- Investigations – blood count, serum chemistry, thyroid function, B_{12} and folate, with other tests as indicated
- Patients at high risk of suicide should be referred to specialist psychiatric services
- In addition, it is recommended that a rating scale be used such as the Hamilton Rating scale for Depression or the Montgomery-Asberg Depression Rating scale be used to assess response to treatment

Treatment modalities and efficacy

Summary of evidence

- Psychoeducation (IIa)
- Physical treatments
  - Antidepressant drugs (Ia)
  - Electroconvulsive therapy (ECT) (Ia)
  - Transcranial Magnetic Stimulation (TMS) (III)
  - Vagal nerve stimulation (VNS) (no evidence in elderly)
- Psychological treatments
  - Supportive (III)
  - Cognitive Behaviour Therapy (CBT) (Ia)
  - Inter-Personal Therapy (IPT) (Ia)
  - Problem-solving therapy (IIb)
  - Family therapy (III)
  - Psychodynamic psychotherapy (Ib)
  - Self-help (IIb)
- Other
  - Light (photo-) therapy (IIb)
  - Exercise (III)
  - Music therapy (III)
  - Herbal (St. John's Wort) (no evidence in elderly)

Treatment in relation to treatment type (Evidence levels Ia–IIa; strength of recommendations A/B)

Type of depression	**Treatment modality**
Psychotic depression	Combined antidepressant or ECT – urgent referral indicated
Severe (non-psychotic depression)	Combined antidepressant and psychological therapy
Moderate depressive episode	Antidepressant *or* psychological therapy (CBT, problem-solving, IPT or brief psychodynamic psychotherapy)
Dysthymia	Antidepressant
Recent onset sub-threshold (minor) depression	Watchful waiting
Persistent sub-threshold (minor) depression	Antidepressant
Grief/bereavement	Treat as for moderate depression if duration and intensity indicate help needed

Considerations in selecting an antidepressant

Factors that matter in choosing an antidepressant

- Age-associated pharmacokinetics (less important for newer antidepressants) (Ia)
- Depression type (e.g. psychotic/non-psychotic) (Ib)
- Prior response to a particular agent (III)
- Tolerability (Ib)
- Safety (Ia)
- Potential side effects (Ia)
- Drug interactions (Ia)
- Likely compliance (IIa)
- Co-morbidity (dementia, physical disorder) (IIa)

Factors that are less important

- Efficacy (all are about equally effective) (Ib)
- Speed of action (all are about the same) (Ib)

Antidepressant drugs in the acute phase of treatment

Summary of evidence

- They are effective in older patients with moderate to severe depressive episode (Ia).
- There are no important differences in speed of onset, although in general older people take longer to recover than younger adults (Ia–IIb)
- Their efficacy in acute minor (subthreshold) depression and uncomplicated grief is unproven (Ib)
- There is some evidence although not extensive that antidepressants may be effective in dysthymia in older people (Ib)

- Antidepressants are effective in patients with a range of physical co-morbid conditions, but tolerability varies (Ia)
- Antidepressants are effective in the treatment of depression associated with dementia (Ib)

Recommendations for practice

- Patients with moderate to severe depressive episode can be successfully treated with an antidepressant drug (A)
- For persistent minor depression (>4 weeks) an antidepressant trial should be considered (B)
- In primary care SSRIs are favoured as the first line of treatment in many developed countries (D)
- Patients with severe depressive episode being treated in psychiatric units should be considered for tricyclic antidepressant treatment (B)
- Older antidepressants should be avoided in patients at risk of suicide (D)
- If an older tricyclic is to be prescribed it is recommended that blood pressure (including postural drop) and an EKG (ECG) be checked (D)
- For patients with moderate to severe depression in dementia treatment with an SSRI, moclobemide or venlafaxine is recommended, along with support to the caregiver (B)
- It is recommended that post-stroke depression be treated with an SSRI (C)
- In patients with co-morbidity the recommended antidepressants are SSRIs, bupropion SR, venlafaxine, mirtazepine and nefazodone (D)
- There is insufficient evidence to recommend low dosage antidepressants in major depression (B)
- In frail patients it is advisable to 'start low, go slow' (D)
- Given the range of antidepressants available it may be advisable to become familiar with one or two agents from the main classes (D)

Patients who do not respond to first-line treatment

Summary of evidence

- Extending the length of trial in partial responders may result in improvement in up to 50% more patients (IIa)
- Switching class from one antidepressant to another is associated with response rates of 50% in uncontrolled series and lower rates in prospective trial data on younger patients (IIb)
- Augmentation with lithium salts may be effective in about 50% of patients – with retrospective studies reporting higher rates than prospective one – but toxicity may occur in 11–23%. Regular blood monitoring is required for lithium (IIb)
- In mixed-aged patients with more rigorously-defined resistant depression both venlafaxine and ECT have been reported to show rates of recovery in between 30 and 50% respectively (IIb)
- Within the emerging concept of vascular depression there is some evidence of a lower response to antidepressant monotherapy but the response rate to ECT may be as favourable as for other patients but with an increased risk of ECT-induced delirium (III)

Recommendations for practice (Level C)

- If little or no response (<25% change in symptoms) by 4 weeks
  - Increase the dose OR if dosage optimal
  - Change to another antidepressant (substitution)
- If partial response (25–50% improvement in symptoms) by 4 weeks:

  –Increase dose (if not already optimal)
  - Continue for further 2–4 weeks
  - Consider augmentation (see text)

- If little further improvement:
  - Augment OR
  - Substitute to another class
- At any stage ECT may be the preferred option
- Psychological treatment may be used adjunctively with some evidence of improved outcome

ECT–indications

- Patient actively suicidal
- Urgent treatment to prevent deterioration in health (including food/fluid refusal)
- Psychotic depression
- Inadequate response to two trials of medication
- Intolerance to medication
- Prior good response

Psychotherapy

Summary of evidence

- The strongest evidence of efficacy exists for CBT and IPT (Ib)
- There is some evidence too of efficacy for brief dynamic psychotherapy, problem-solving therapy and life review (Ib–IIa)
- Psychotherapy is effective as a main treatment for older patients with moderate major depressive episode (Ib)
- It is effective when combined with medication in severe major depression and the combination is more effective than either modality alone (Ib)
- Problem-solving therapy may be an effective treatment for subthreshold (minor) depression but only when the personnel delivering it have been trained to a consistent level (Ib)

- Offering support to patients and their caregivers is not the same as doing nothing. Simple support is associated with fairly high rates of symptom resolution in mild depression (Ib).
- A structured family intervention to caregivers of people with dementia has been shown to reduce depressive symptoms (Ib)

Recommendations for practice

- It is recommended that primary care teams treating elderly depressed patients have access to personnel with training in either CBT or IPT (A)
- Wherever possible supportive care should be offered to the patient and, where relevant, caregiver (B)
- It is recommended that psychological interventions are available to patients with mild to moderate major depressive episode as a first choice treatment (A)

Collaborative care

Summary of evidence

- Passive feedback of screening results, distributing guidelines and other educational material to primary care physicians are ineffective on their own (Ib)
- Shared care of depressive disorder has been shown to be effective in primary care and care homes for older and mixed-aged patients (Ib)
- Compliance with medication improves with shared care for younger depressed patients (Ib) and there is some positive evidence too in older depressed patients (IIa)

Recommendations for practice (level B)

There is insufficient evidence to recommend any one particular model but the following are successful:

- Identifying a care co-ordinator (case manager),
- Active follow-up of patients,
- Giving educational packages to caregivers (in residential and nursing homes) and
- Enhancing the links between primary and secondary care are successful components

Continuation and maintenance treatment

Summary of evidence

- Current evidence suggests a continuation period for major depressive episode of 12 months for a first episode; longer for a recurrent disorder (Ib)
- There is little available evidence regarding non-major depression
- Effective maintenance for the prevention of recurrence has been demonstrated for nortriptyline, dosulepin, citalopram and paroxetine (Ib)
- There is a lack of consensus on how long maintenance treatment should last or whether it should last for life (IV)

Recommendations for practice

- On current evidence patients with a first onset major depression should be continued on the same dosage of antidepressant that improved them for 12 months (B)
- Those with recurrent depression should be continued at the same dosage that improved them, with a review held at 12 months with the patient to discuss risk factors (C)
- For high risk patients, treatment should be continued for at least 3 years or indefinitely (C)

When to refer the patient for specialist advice

- When the diagnosis in doubt
- When depression is severe, as evidenced by;
  - Psychotic depression
  - Severe risk to health because of failure to eat or drink
  - Suicide risk
- Complex therapy is indicated (for example in cases with medical co-morbidity)
- When first-line therapy fails (although more experienced physicians may wish to pursue a second course of a different antidepressant)

General prognosis

Summary of evidence

- The outcome of depressive disorder in older people is as good as in other age groups (Ia)
- There may be more susceptibility to relapse (more 'brittle' outcomes) in older patients, although relapse can respond to treatment (Ib)
- The risk of relapse and recurrence can be reduced by antidepressant medication or IPT or a combination of both (Ib)
- The prognosis in patients in the community and in medical wards is much worse and the reasons for this are unclear (Ia)
- Prognostic factors may be divided into clinical features and more general factors (III):
  - Clinical features: slower initial recovery; more severe initial depression; duration >2 years; three or more previous episodes (for recurrence); previous history of dysthymia; psychotic symptoms; marked initial anxiety; extensive deep white matter and basal ganglia grey matter brain disease; cognitive impairment
  - General factors: chronic stress associated with poor environment, crime and poverty; a new physical illness or worsening of a physical illness; becoming a victim of crime; poor perceived (but not necessarily tangible) social support

Recommendations for practice

- It is recommended that major depression in older people be treated like other chronic disabling conditions, with attention to follow-up after recovery in the acute phase (C)
- It is recommended that patients who present with cognitive impairment when depressed (e.g. MMSE score below 24) be followed up for later signs of dementia (C)

Suicide

Summary of evidence

- It is hard to predict which patients may attempt suicide but there is growing evidence that identifying and managing depressive disorder in primary care is the most effective way to reduce suicide in older people (IV)
- The risk of suicide in older people can be divided into general factors and clinical features (IIa):
  - *General factors*: greater age (>80); male gender; living alone; inadequate social support; significant loss; alcohol abuse (not specific to elderly); cultural acceptability (in some societies more acceptable than others);
  - *Psychiatric factors*: past attempt; marked psychomotor agitation; insomnia; severe guilt; hopelessness; persistent hypochondriasis; suicidal ideation.

Recommendations for practice

Until more definitive evidence becomes available, it is recommended that the most likely strategy to impact on suicide rates is the effective identification and management of depressive disorder in primary care (D)

Prevention of relapse and recurrence

Recommendations for prevention of relapse

- Treat acute phase to remission of *all* symptoms (not elderly-specific) (A)
- Continue antidepressants for at last 12 months (new case) or longer (recurrent case) (B)
- For major depressive disorder where possible combine pharmacological treatment with psychological therapy (B)
- Follow-up patients where possible (C)

Recommendations for prevention of recurrence

- Identify patients at high risk of recurrence and treat with medication (SSRI or tricyclic) and/or psychological treatment (A)
- Consider maintenance ECT for high risk cases (C)
- Follow-up patients systematically where possible (C)

appendix A

Strategic references used in the evidence base

Alexopoulos GS, Katz IR, Reynolds CF, Carpenter D, Docherty JP. (2001) The expert consensus guideline series: Pharmacotherapy of Depressive Disorders in Older Patients. *Postgrad Med Special Report.* (October):1–86, Expert Knowledge Systems, LLC, McGraw-Hill Healthcare Information Programs, Minneapolis, US. **[EXP]**

Anderson IM, Nutt DJ, Deakin JFW. (2000) Evidence-based guidelines for treating depressive disorders with antidepressants: a revision of the British Association for Psychopharmacology guidelines. *Journal of Psychopharmacology* **14**:3020. **[BAP]**

Chiu E, Ames D, Draper B, Sowdon J. (1999) Depressive disorders in the elderly: a review. In: Maj M, Sartorius N, eds. *Depressive Disorders*. Chichester: John Wiley & Sons, 313–63. **[WPA]**

Lebowitz BD, Pearson JL, Schneider LS et al. (1997) Diagnosis and treatment of depression in late life. *Journal of the American Medical Association* **278**:1186–90. **[NIH]**

NIH Consensus Panel. (1992) Diagnosis and treatment of depression in late life. *Journal of the American Medical Association* **268**:1018–24. **[NIH]**

Schneider LS, Reynolds CF III, Lebowitz BD, Friedhoff AJ. (1991) *Diagnosis and Treatment of Depression in Late Life*. Washington, DC: American Psychiatric Press. **[NIH]**

Shekelle PG, Woolf SH, Eccles M, Grimshaw M. (1999) Developing guidelines. *British Medical Journal* **318**:593–6.

World Psychiatric Association. (1999) WPA International Committee for Prevention and Treatment of Depression. *Depressive Disorders in Older Persons*. New York: NCM Publishers. **[PTD]** Available online: http://www.wpanet.org/sectorial/edu4.

appendix B

General references

Abramson J, Berger A, Krumholz HM, Vaccarino V. (2001) Depression and risk of heart failure among older persons with isolated systolic hypertension. *Archives of Internal Medicine* **161**:1725–30.

Aguglia, E. (2000) Reboxetine in the maintenance therapy of depressive disorder in the elderly: a long-term open study. *International Journal of Geriatric Psychiatry* **15**:784–93.

Alexopoulos GS, Abrams RC, Young RC, Shamoian CA. (1988) Cornell Scale for depression in dementia. *Biological Psychiatry* **23**:271–84.

Alexopoulos GS, Meyers BS, Young RC, Campbell S, Silbersweig D, Charlson M. (1997) 'Vascular depression' hypothesis. *Archives of General Psychiatry* **54**:915–22.

Allen NHP, Burns A. (1995) The non-cognitive features of dementia. *Reviews in Clinical Gerontology* **5**:57–75.

Almeida OP, Almeida SA. (1999) Short versions of the geriatric depression scale: a study of their validity for the diagnosis of a major depressive episode according to ICD-10 and DSM-IV. *International Journal of Geriatric Psychiatry* **14**:858–65.

Andersen G, Vestergaard K, Lauritzen L. (1994) Effective treatment of post-stroke depression with the selective serotonin reuptake inhibitor citalopram. *Stroke* **25**:1099–104.

Andersson S, Krogstad JM, Finset A. (1999) Apathy and depressed mood in acquired brain damage: relationship to lesion localisation and psychophysiological reactivity. *Psychological Medicine* **29**:447–56.

Andreoli V, Carbognin G, Abati A, Vantini G. (1999) Reboxetine in the treatment of depression in the elderly. *Journal of Geriatric Psychiatry & Neurology* **12**:206–10.

Arean PA, Perri MG, Nezu AM, Schein RL, Christopher F, Joseph TX. (1993) Comparative effectiveness of social problem-solving therapy and reminiscence therapy as treatment for depression in older adults. *Journal of Consulting and Clinical Psychology* **61**:1003–10.

Ariyo AA, Haan M, Tangen CM et al. (2000) Depressive symptoms and risks of coronary heart disease and mortality in elderly Americans. Cardiovascular Health Study Collaborative Research Group. *Circulation* **102**:1773–9.

Arve S, Tilvis RS, Lehtonen A, Valvanne J, Sairanen S. (1999) Coexistence of lowered mood and cognitive impairment of elderly people in five birth cohorts. *Aging* **11**:90–5.

Ashtari M, Greenwald BS, Kramer-Ginsberg E et al. (1999) Hippocampal/amygdala volumes in geriatric depression. *Psychological Medicine* **29**:629–38.

Avery D, Winokur G. (1976) Mortality in depressed patients treated with electroconvulsive therapy and antidepressants. *Archives of General Psychiatry* **33**:1029–37.

Baldwin RC. (2000) Poor prognosis of depression in elderly people: causes and actions. *Annals of Medicine* **32**:252–6.

Banerjee S et al. (1996) Randomized controlled trial of effect of intervention by psychogeriatric teams on depression in frail elderly people at home. *British Medical Journal* **313**:1058–61.

Barraclough BM. (1971) Suicide in the elderly. *British Journal of Psychiatry* (special suppl 6):87–97.

Bartels SJ, Forester B, Miles KM, Joyce T. (2000) Mental health service use by elderly patients with bipolar disorder and unipolar depression. *American Journal of Geriatric Psychiatry* **8**:160–6.

Beekman AT, Copeland JR, Prince MJ. (1999) Review of community prevalence of depression in later life. *British Journal of Psychiatry* **174**:307–11.

Benazzi F. (2000) Late-life chronic depression: a 399-case study in private practice. *International Journal of Geriatric Psychiatry* **15**:1–6.

Black SA, Markides KS, Miller TQ. (1998) Correlates of depressive symptomatology among older community-dwelling Mexican Americans: the Hispanic EPESE. *Journal of Gerontology Series B – Psychological Sciences* **53**:S198–208.

Black SA. (1999) Increased health burden associated with comorbid depression in older diabetic Mexican Americans. Results from the Hispanic Established Population for the Epidemiologic Study of the Elderly Survey. *Diabetes Care* **22**:56–64.

Blank K, Robison J, Doherty E, Prigerson H, Duffy J, Schwartz HI. (2001) Life-sustaining treatment and assisted death choices in depressed older patients. *Journal of the American Geriatric Society* **49**:153–61.

Blazer D. (1991) Clinical features of depression in old age: a case for minor depression. *Current Opinion in Psychiatry* **4**:596–9.

Bowskill RJ, Bridges PK (1997) Treatment-resistant affective disorders. *British Journal of Hospital Medicine* **57**:171–2.

Braam AW, Sonnenberg CM, Beekman AT, Deeg DL, van Tilburg W. (2000) Religious denomination as a symptom-formation factor of depression in older Dutch citizens. *International Journal of Geriatric Psychiatry* **15**:458–66.

Breuer B, Anderson R. (2000) The relationship of tamoxifen with dementia, depression and dependence in activities of daily living in elderly nursing home residents. *Women & Health* **31**:71–85.

Brodaty H, Hickie I, Mason C, Prenter L. (2000) A prospective follow-up study of ECT outcome in older depressed patients. *Journal of Affective Disorders* **60**:101–11.

Brodaty H, Luscombe G, Parker G et al. (2001) Early and late onset depression in old age: different aetiologies, same phenomenology. *Journal of Affective Disorders* **66**:225–36.

Brown GK, Bruce ML, Pearson JL and the PROSPECT Study Group. (2001) High-risk management guidelines for elderly suicidal patients in primary care. *International Journal of Geriatric Psychiatry* **16**:593–601.

Bump GM, Mulsant BH, Pollock BG et al. (2001) Paroxetine versus nortriptyline in the continuation and maintenance treatment of depression in the elderly. *Depression & Anxiety* **13**:38–44.

Burns A, Lawlor B, Craig S. (1999) *Assessment Scales in Old Age Psychiatry*. Martin Dunitz, London.

Bush BA. (1999) Major life events as risk factors for post-stroke depression. *Brain Injury* **13**:131–7.

Caine ED. (2001) Presentation of the Joint Meeting of the International Psychogeriatric Association and the Faculty of Psychiatry of Old Age and Australian and New Zealand College of Psychiatrists; Lorne, Victoria, Australia (Abstract p.30).

Carson AJ, MacHale S, Allen K et al. (2000) Depression after stroke and lesion location: a systematic review. *Lancet* **356**:122–6.

Cattell H, Jolley DJ. (1995) One hundred cases of suicide in elderly people. *British Journal of Psychiatry* **166**:451–7.

Chou KL, Chi I. (2000) Stressful life events and depressive symptoms among old women and men: a longitudinal study. *Journal of Aging and Human Development* **51**:275–93.

Cole MG, Bellavance F. (1997a) The prognosis of depression in old age. *American Journal of Psychiatry* **5**:4–14.

Cole MG, Bellavance F. (1997b) Depression in elderly medical inpatients: a meta-analysis of outcomes. *Canadian Medical Association Journal* **157**:1055–60.

Cole MG, Elie LM, McCusker J, Bellavance F, Mansour A. (2000) Feasibility and effectiveness of treatments for depression in elderly medical inpatients: a systematic review. *International Psychogeriatrics* **12**:453–61.

Cole MG, Yaffe MJ. (1996) Pathway to psychiatric care of the elderly with depression. *International Journal of Geriatric Psychiatry* **11**:157–61.

Conwell Y, Lyness JM, Duberstein P et al. (2000) Completed suicide among older patients in primary care practices: a controlled study. *Journal of the American Geriatrics Society* 4823–9.

Copeland JRM, Beekman ATF, Dewey ME et al. (1999) Depression in Europe: geographical distribution among older people. *British Journal of Psychiatry* **174**:312–21.

Cronin-Stubbs D, de Leon CF, Beckett LA, Filed TS, Glynn RJ, Evans DA. (2000) Six-year effect of depressive symptoms on the course of physical disability in community-living older adults. *Archives of Internal Medicine* **160**:3074–80.

Cuijpers PIM. (1998) Psychological outreach programmes for the depressed elderly: a meta-analysis of effects and dropouts. *International Journal Geriatric Psychiatry* **13**:41–8.

Dentino AN, Pieper CF, Rao MK et al. (1999) Association of interleukin-6 and other biologic variables with depression in older people living in the community. *Journal of the American Geriatrics Society* **47**:6–11.

Dhondt ADF, Hooijer C. (1995) Iatrogenic origins of depression in the elderly. *International Journal of Geriatric Psychiatry* **10**:1–8.

Duberstein PR, Conwell Y, Seidlitz L, Lyness JM, Cox C, Caine ED. (1999) Age and suicidal ideation in older depressed inpatients. *American Journal of Geriatric Psychiatry* **7**:289–96.

Dwyer M, Byrne GJ. (2000) Disruptive vocalization and depression in older nursing home residents. *International Psychogeriatrics* **12**:463–71.

Dyer CB, Pavlik VN, Murphy KP, Hyman DJ. (2000) The high prevalence of depression and dementia in elder abuse or neglect. *Journal of the American Geriatrics Society* **48**:205–8.

Evans M, Hammond M, Wilson K et al. (1997) Placebo-controlled treatment trial of depression in elderly physically ill patients. *International Journal of Geriatric Psychiatry* **12**:817–24.

Flint AJ, Rifat SL. (2000) Maintenance treatment for recurrent depression in late life: a four year outcome study. *American Journal of Geriatric Psychiatry* **8**:112–16.

Folstein MF, Folstein SE, McHugh PR. (1975) 'Mini-Mental State': a practical method for grading the cognitive state of patients for the clinician. *Journal of Psychiatric Research* **12**:189–98.

Forsell Y, Winblad E. (1998) Feelings of anxiety and associated variables in a very elderly population. *International Journal of Geriatric Psychiatry* **13**:454–8.

Forsen L, Meyer HE, Sogaard AJ, Naess S, Schei B, Edna TH. (1999) Mental distress and risk of hip fracture: Do broken hearts lead to broken bones? *Journal of Epidemiology & Community Health* **53**:343–7.

Galaria II, Casten RJ, Rovner BW. (2000) Development of a shorter version of the geriatric depression scale for visually impaired older patients. *International Psychogeriatrics* **12**:435–43.

Gallo JJ, Ryan SD, Ford DE. (1999) Attitudes, knowledge, and behavior of family physicians regarding depression in late life. *Archives of Family Medicine* **8**:249–56.

Gatz M, Fiske A, Fox LS et al. (1998) Empirically validated psychological treatments for older adults. *Journal of Mental Health and Aging* **4**:9–46.

Gerson S, Belin TR, Kaufman A, Mintz J, Jarvik L. (1999) Pharmacological and psychological treatments for depressed older patients: a meta-analysis and overview of recent findings. *Harvard Review of Psychiatry* **7**:1–28.

Gill D, Hatcher S. (1999) Antidepressant drugs in depressed patients who also have a physical illness (Cochrane Review). In: *The Cochrane Library*, Issue 3, Oxford: Update Software.

Gonzalez HM, Haan MN, Hinton L. (2001) Acculturation and the prevalence of depression in older Mexican Americans: baseline results of the Sacramento Area Latino Study on Aging. *Journal of the American Geriatrics Society* **49**:948–53.

Guelfi JD, Bouhassira M, Bonett-Perrin E, Lancrenon S. (1999) The study of efficacy of fluoxetine versus tianeptine in the treatment of elderly depressed patients followed in general practice. *Encephale* **25**:265–70.

Guscott R, Grof P. (1991) The clinical meaning of refractory depression: a review for the clinician. *American Journal of Psychiatry* **148**:695–704.

Gustafson Y, Nilsson I, Mattsson M et al. (1995) Epidemiology and treatment of post-stroke depression. *Drugs and Aging* **7**:298–309.

Hamalainen J, Kaprio J, Isometsa E et al. (2001) Cigarette smoking, alcohol intoxication and major depressive episode in a representative population sample. *Journal of Epidemiology & Community Health* **55**:573–6.

Hamilton M. (1960) A rating scale for depression. *Journal of Neurology, Neurosurgery and Psychiatry* **23**:56–62.

Harris T, Brown GW, Robinson R. (1999) Befriending as an intervention for chronic depression among women in an inner city. 2: Role of fresh-start experiences and baseline psychosocial factors in remission from depression. *British Journal of Psychiatry* **174**:225–32.

Harwood D, Hawton K, Hope T, Jacob R. (2001) Psychiatric disorder and personality factors associated with suicide in older people: a descriptive and case-control study. *International Journal of Geriatric Psychiatry* **16**:155–65.

Helm HM, Hays JC, Flint EP, Koenig HG, Blazer DG. (2000) Does private religious activity prolong survival? *Journal of Gerontology Series A – Biological Sciences & Medical Sciences* **55**:M400–5.

Henderson AS, Jorm AF, Korten AE, Jacomb P, Christensen H, Rodgers B. (1998) Symptoms of depression and anxiety during adult life: evidence of a decline in prevalence with age. *Psychological Medicine* **28**:1321–8.

Holmes JD, House AO. (2000) Psychiatric illness after hip fracture. *Age & Ageing* **29**:537–46.

Hoyl MT, Alessi CA, Harker JO. (1999) Development and testing of a five item version of the Geriatric Depression Scale. *Journal of the American Geriatric Society* **47**:873–78.

Huang BY, Comoni-Huntley J, Hays JC, Huntley RR, Galanos AN, Blazer DG. (2000) Impact of depressive symptoms on hospitalisation risk in community-dwelling older persons. *Journal of the American Geriatrics Society* **48**:1279–84.

Ingold BB, Yersin B, Wietlisbach V, Burckhardt P, Bumand B, Bula CJ. (2000) Characteristics associated with inappropriate hospital use in elderly patients admitted to a general internal medicine service. *Aging* **12**:430–8.

Jonas BS, Mussolino ME. (2000) Symptoms of depression as prospective risk factor for stroke. *Psychosomatic Medicine* **62**:463–71.

Jorm AF. (2001) Association of hypotension with positive and negative affect and depressive symptoms in the elderly. *British Journal of Psychiatry* **178**:553–5.

Kaplan MS, Adamek ME, Rhoades JA. (1998) Prevention of suicide. Physicians' assessment of firearm availability. *American Journal of Preventive Medicine* **15**:60–4.

Katona C, Livingston G. (2000) Impact of screening of old people with physical illness for depression? *Lancet* **356**:91–2.

Katzman R, Brown T, Fuld P, Peck A, Schechter R, Schimmel H. (1983) Validation of a short orientation-memory-concentration test of cognitive impairment. *American Journal of Psychiatry* **140**:734–9.

Keller MB, Boland RJ. (1998) Implications of failing to achieve successful long-term maintenance treatment of recurrent unipolar depression. *Biological Psychiatry* **44**:348–60.

Kiosses DN, Alexopoulos GS, Murphy C. (2000) Symptoms of striatofrontal dysfunction contribute to disability in geriatric depression. *International Journal of Geriatric Psychiatry* **15**:992–9.

Kirby D, Ames D. (2001) Hyponatraemia and selective serotonin re-uptake inhibitors in elderly patients. *International Journal of Geriatric Psychiatry* **16**:484–93.

Kirby M, Bruce I, Coakley D, Lawlor BA. (1999a) Dysthymia among the community-dwelling elderly. *International Journal of Geriatric Psychiatry* **14**:440–5.

Kirby M, Denihan A, Bruce I, Radic A, Coakley D, Lawlor BA. (1999b) Influence of symptoms of anxiety on treatment of depression in later life in primary care: questionnaire survey. *British Medical Journal* **318**:579–80.

Kritz-Silverstein D, Barrett-Conor E, Corbeau C. (2001) Cross-sectional and prospective study of exercise and depressed mood in the elderly: the Rancho Bernardo study. *American Journal of Epidemiology* **153**:596–603.

Kurlowicz LH. (2001) Benefits of psychiatric consultation-liaison nurse interventions for older hospitalized patients and their nurses. *Archives of Psychiatric Nursing* **15**:53–61.

Laidlaw K. (2001) An empirical review of cognitive therapy for late life depression: does research suggest adaptations are necessary for cognitive therapy with older adults? *Clinical Psychology and Psychotherapy* **8**:1–14.

Lampinen P, Heikkinen RL, Ruoppila I. (2000) Changes in intensity of physical exercise as predictors depressive symptoms among older adults an eight-year follow-up. *Preventive Medicine* **30**:371–80.

Lenze EJ, Miller MD, Dew MA et al. (2001a) Subjective health measures and acute treatment outcomes in geriatric depression. *International Journal of Psychiatry* **16**:1149–55.

Lenze EJ, Rogers JC, Martire LM et al. (2001b) The association of late-life depression and anxiety with physical disability: a review of the literature and prospectus for future research. *American Journal of Geriatric Psychiatry* **9**:113–35.

Lifton I, Kett PA. (2000) Suicidal ideation and the choice of advance directives by elderly persons with affective disorder. *Psychiatric Services* **51**:1447–9.

Little JT, Reynolds CF III, Dew MA et al. (1998) How common is resistance to treatment in recurrent, nonpsychotic geriatric depression? *American Journal of Psychiatry* **155**:1035–8.

Livingston G, Yard P, Beard A, Katona C. (2000) A nurse-coordinated educational initiative addressing primary care professionals' attitudes to and problem-solving in depression in older people – a pilot study. *International Journal of Geriatric Psychiatry* **15**:401–5.

Llewellyn-Jones RH, Baikie KA, Smithers H, Cohen J, Snowdon J, Tennant C. (1999) Multifaceted shared care intervention for late-life depression in residential care randomized controlled trial. *British Medical Journal* **319**:676–82.

Lyness JM, Caine ED, King DA, Conwell Y, Cox C, Duberstein PR. (1999a) Cerebrovascular risk factors and depression in older primary care patients: testing a vascular brain disease model of depression. *American Journal of Geriatric Psychiatry* **7**:252–8.

Lyness JM, King DA, Cox C, Yoediono Z, Caine ED. (1999b) The importance of subsyndromal depression in older primary care patients: prevalence and associated functional disability. *Journal of the American Geriatric Society* **47**:647–52.

Mackinnon A, McCallum J, Andrews G, Anderson I. (1998) The Center For Epidemiological Studies Depression Scale in older samples in Indonesia, North Korea, Myanmar, Sri Lanka, and Thailand. *Journal of Gerontology B – Psychological Sciences* **53**:343–52.

Marraccini RL, Reynolds CF III, Houck PR et al. (1999) A double-blind, placebo-controlled assessment of nortriptyline's side effects during 3-year maintenance treatment in elderly patients with recurrent major depression. *International Journal of Geriatric Psychiatry* **14**:1014–18.

Marriott A, Donaldson C, Tarrier N, Burns A. (2000) Effectiveness of cognitive–behavioural family intervention in reducing the burden of care in carers of patients with Alzheimer's disease. *British Journal of Psychiatry* **176**:557–62.

McCurren C, Dowe D, Rattle D, Looney S. (1999) Depression among nursing home residents: testing an intervention strategy. *Applied Nursing Research* **12**:185–95.

McCusker J, Cole M, Keller E, Bellavance F, Berard A. (1998) Effectiveness of treatments of depression in older ambulatory patients. *Archives of International Medicine* **158**:705–12.

Meldon SW, Emerman CL, Moffa DA, Schubert DS. (1999) Utility of clinical characteristics in identifying depression in geriatric ED patients. *American Journal of Emergency Medicine* **17**:522–5.

Mittman N, Herrmann N, Einarson TR et al. (1997) The efficacy, safety and tolerability of antidepressants in late life depression: a meta-analysis. *Journal of Affective Disorders* **46**:191–217.

Montgomery SA, Asberg M. (1979) A new depression scale designed to be sensitive to change. *British Journal of Psychiatry* **134**:382–9.

Morgan K, Bath PA. (1998) Customary physical activity and psychological wellbeing: a longitudinal study. *Age & Ageing* **27**(suppl 3):35–40.

Mossey JM, Knott KA, Higgins M, Talerico K. (1996) Effectiveness of a psychosocial intervention, interpersonal counseling, for subdysthymic depression in medically ill elderly. *Journal of Gerontology: Medical Sciences* **51A**:M172–M178.

Mottram P, Wilson K, Copeland J. (2000) Validation of the Hamilton Depression Scale and Montgomery and Asberg rating scales in terms of AGECAT depression cases. *International Journal of Geriatric Psychiatry* **15**:1113–19.

Moussaoui D. (1999) Depression in the elderly 1 (editorial). *WPA Bulletin on Depression* **4**:2.

Mulsant BH, Alexopoulos GS, Reynolds CF III et al and the PROSPECTS Study Group. (2001) Pharmacological treatment of depression in older primary care patients: the PROSPECT algorithm. *International Journal of Geriatric Psychiatry* **16**:585–92.

Nobler MS, Pelton GH, Sackeim HA. (1999) Cerebral blood flow and metabolism in late-life depression. *Journal of Geriatric Psychiatry & Neurology* **12**:118–27.

Nyth AL, Gottries CG, Lyby K et al. (1992) A multicenter clinical study of citalopram and placebo in elderly depressed patients with and without concomitant dementia. *Acta Psychiatrica Scandinavica* **86**:138–45.

O'Brien J, Ames D, Chiu E, Schweitzer I, Desmond P, Tress B. (1998) Severe deep white matter lesions and outcome in elderly patients with major depressive disorder: follow-up study. *British Medical Journal* **317**:982–4.

O'Brien JT, Ames D. (1994) Why do the depressed elderly die? *International Journal of Geriatric Psychiatry* **9**:689–93.

Ohira T, Iso H, Sankai T et al. (2001) Prospective study of depressive symptoms and risk of stroke among Japanese. *Stroke* **32**:903–8.

Old Age Depression Interest Group (1993) How long should the elderly take antidepressants? A double blind placebo-controlled study of continuation/prophylaxis therapy with dothiepin. *British Journal of Psychiatry* **162**:175–82.

Palsson S, Johansson B, Berg S, Skoog I. (2000) A population study on the influence of depression on neuropsychological functioning in 85-year-olds. *Acta Psychiatrica Scandinavica* **101**:185–93.

Penninx BW, Deeg DJ, van Eijk JT, Beekman AT, Gurainik JM. (2000) Changes in depression and physical decline in older adults: a longitudinal perspective. *Journal of Affective Disorders* **61**:1–12.

Penninx BW, Guralnik JM, Pahor M et al. (1998) Chronically depressed mood and cancer risk in older persons. *Journal of the National Cancer Institute* **90**:1888–93.

Peveler R, Kendrick T (2001) Treatment delivery and guidelines in primary care. *British Medical Bulletin* **57**:193–206.

Pinquart M, Sorensen S. (2001) How effective are psychotherapeutic and other psychosocial interventions with older adults? A meta-analysis. *Journal of Mental Health and Aging* **7**:207–43.

Prince MJ, Harwood RH, Thomas A, Mann AH. (1998) A prospective population-based cohort study of the effects of disablement and social milieu on the onset and maintenance of late-life depression. The Gospel Oak Project VII. *Psychological Medicine* **28**:337–50.

Proctor R, Burns A, Stratton Powell H et al. (1999) Behavioural management in nursing and residential homes: a randomised controlled trial. *Lancet* 1999; **354**:26–9.

Rabins PV, Black BS, Roca R et al. (2000) Effectiveness of a nurse-based outreach program for identifying and treating psychiatric illness in the elderly. *Journal of the American Medical Association* **283**:2802–9.

Rait G, Burns A, Baldwin R et al. (1999) Screening for depression in African-Caribbean elders. *Family Practice* **16**:591–5.

Rao V, Lyketsos CG. (2000) The benefits and risks of ECT for patients with primary dementia who also suffer from depression. *International Journal of Geriatric Psychiatry* **15**:729–35.

Reynolds CF III, Frank E, Perel JM et al. (1999a) Nortriptyline and interpersonal psychotherapy as maintenance therapies for recurrent major depression: a randomized controlled trial in patients older than 59 years. *Journal of the American Medical Association* **281**:39–45.

Reynolds CF III, Miller MD, Pasternak RE et al. (1999b) Treatment of bereavement-related major depressive episodes in later life: a controlled study of acute and continuation treatment with nortriptyline and interpersonal psychotherapy. *American Journal of Psychiatry* **156**:202 8.

Ritchie K, Touchon J, Ledesert B. (1998) Progressive disability in senile dementia is accelerated in the presence of depression. *International Journal of Geriatric Psychiatry* **13**:459–61.

Robinson RG, Chemerinski E, Jorge R. (1999) Pathophysiology of secondary depressions in the elderly. *Journal of Geriatric Psychiatry & Neurology* **12**:128–36.

Rojas-Fernandez C, Thomas VS, Carver D, Tonks R. (1999) Suboptimal use of antidepressant in the elderly: a population-based study in Nova Scotia. *Clinical Therapeutics* **21**:1937–50.

Romach MK, Sproule BA, Sellers EM, Somer G, Busto UE. (1999) Long-term codeine use is associated with depressive symptoms. *Journal of Clinical Psychopharmacology* **19**:373–6.

Roose SP, Suthers KM. (1998) Antidepressant response in late-life depression. *Journal of Clinical Psychiatry* 59(suppl 10):4–8.

Rosen J, Mulsant BH, Pollock BG. (2000) Sertraline in the treatment of minor depression in nursing home residents: a pilot study. *International Journal of Geriatric Psychiatry* **15**:177–80.

Rosen J, Rogers JC, Marin RS, Mulsant BH, Shahar A, Reynolds CF III. (1997) Control-relevant intervention in the treatment of minor and major depression in a long-term care facility. *American Journal of Geriatric Psychiatry* **5**:247–57.

Roth M, Mountjoy CQ, Amrein R. (1996) Moclobemide in elderly patients with cognitive decline and depression: an international double-blind placebo-controlled study. *British Journal of Psychiatry* **168**:149–57.

Rutz W, yon Knorring L, Walinder J. (1989) Frequency of suicide on Gotland after systematic postgraduate education of general practitioners. *Acta Psychiatric Scandinavia* **80**:151–4.

Salvatore T. (2000) Elder suicide: a preventable tragedy. *Caring* **19**:34–7.

Schoevers RA, Beekkman AT, Deeg DJ, Geerlings MI, Jonker C, van Tilberg W. (2000) Risk factors for depression in later life: results of a prospective community-based study (AMSTEL). *Journal of Affective Disorders* **59**:127–37.

Scogin F, McElreath L. (1994) Efficacy of psychosocial treatments for geriatric depression: a quantitative review. *Journal of Consulting Clinical Psychology* **62**:69–74.

Shibata H, Kumagai S, Watanabe S, Suzuki T. (1999) Relationship of serum cholesterols and vitamin E to depressive states in the elderly. *Journal of Epidemiology* **9**:261–7.

Shmuely Y, Baumgarten M, Rovner B, Berlin J. (2001) Predictors of improvement in health-related quality of life among elderly patients with depression. *International Psychogeriatrics* **13**:63–73.

Simpson SW, Jackson A, Baldwin RC, Burns A. (1997) Subcortical hyperintensities in late-life depression: acute response to treatment and neuropsychological impairment. *International Psychogeriatrics* **9**:257–75.

Snowdon J. (2001) Is depression more prevalent in old age? *Australian and New Zealand Journal of Psychiatry* **35**:782–7.

Stage KB, Bech P, Kragh-Sorensen P, Nair NP, Katona C. (2001) Differences in symptomatology and diagnostic profile in younger and elderly depressed inpatients. *Journal of Affective Disorders* **64**:239–48.

Steffens DC, Byrum CE, McQuoid DR et al. (2000) Hippocampal volume in geriatric depression. *Biological Psychiatry* **48**:301–9.

Steffens DC, Doraiswamy PM, McQuoid DR. (2001) Bupropion SR in the naturalistic treatment of elderly patients with major depression. *International Journal of Geriatric Psychiatry* **16**:862–5.

Steffens DC, Helms MJ, Krishnan KR, Burke GL. (1999) Cerebrovascular disease and depression symptoms in the cardiovascular health study. *Stroke* **30**:2159–66.

Stevens T, Katona C, Manela M, Watkin V, Livingston G. (1999) Drug treatment of older people with affective disorders in the community: lessons from an attempted drug trial. *International Journal of Geriatric Psychiatry* **14**:467–72.

Stroup-Benham CA, Markides KS, Black SA, Goodwin JS. (2000) Relationship between low blood pressure and depressive symptomatology in older people. *Journal of the American Geriatric Society* **48**:250–5.

Sullivan MD, Kempen GI, van Sonderen E, Ormel J. (2000) Models of health-related quality of life in a population of community-dwelling Dutch elderly. *Quality of Life Research* **9**:801–10.

Sutcliffe C, Cordingley L, Burns A et al. (2000) A new version of the Geriatric Depression Scale for nursing and residential home populations: the Geriatric Depression Scale (Residential) (GDS-12R). *International Psychogeriatrics* **12**:173–81.

Tan RSH, Barlow RJ, Abel C et al. (1994) The effect of low dose lofepramine in depressed elderly patients in general medical wards. *British Journal of Clinical Pharmacology* **37**:321–4.

Tannock C, Katona C. (1995) Minor depression in the aged: concepts, prevalence and optimal management. *Drug Therapy* **6**:278–92.

Taylor MP, Reynolds CF III, Frank E et al. (1999) Which elderly depressed patients remain well on maintenance interpersonal psychotherapy alone? Report from the Pittsburgh study of maintenance therapies in late-life depression. *Depression & Anxiety* **10**:55–60.

Tew JD Jr, Mulsant BH, Haskett RF et al. (1999) Acute efficacy of ECT in the treatment of major depression in the Old-Old. *American Journal of Psychiatry* **156**:1865–70.

Thase ME, Rush AJ. (1997) When at first you don't succeed: sequential strategies for antidepressant nonresponders. *Journal of Clinical Psychiatry* **58** (suppl 13):23–9.

Thompson C, Syddall H, Rodin I, Osmond C, Barker DJP. (2001a) Birth weight and the risk of depressive disorder in late life. *British Journal of Psychiatry* **179**:450 5.

Thompson LW, Coon DW, Gallagher-Thompson D, Sommer BR, Koin D. (2001b) Comparison of desipramine and cognitive/behavioral therapy in the treatment of elderly outpatients with mild-to-moderate depression. *American Journal of Geriatric Psychiatry* **9**:225–40.

Trappler B, Cohen CI. (1998) Use of SSRIs in 'very old' depressed nursing home residents. *American Journal of Geriatric Psychiatry* **6**:83–9.

Tuma TA. (2000) Outcome of hospital-treated depression at 4.5 years. An elderly and a younger adult cohort compared. *British Journal of Psychiatry* **176**:224–8.

Turvey CL, Carney C, Arndt S, Wallace RB, Herzog R. (1999) Conjugal loss and syndromal depression in a sample of elders aged 70 years and older. *American Journal of Psychiatry* **156**:1596–601.

van Grootheest DS, Beekman AT, Broese van Groenou MI, Deeg DJ. (1999) Sex differences in depression after widowhood. Do men suffer more? *Social Psychiatry & Psychiatric Epidemiology* **34**:391–8.

von Korff M, Goldberg D. (2001) Improving outcomes in depression. *British Medical Journal* **323**:948–9.

Wallsten SM, Tweed DL, Blazer DG, George LK. (1999) Disability and depressive symptoms in the elderly: the effects of instrumental support and its subjective appraisal. *International Journal of Aging and Human Development* **48**:145–59.

Wang SJ, Liu HC, Fuh JL, Liu CY, Wang PN, Lu SR. (1999) Comorbidity of headaches and depression in the elderly. *Pain* **82**:239–43.

Waterreus A, Blonchard M, Mann A. (1994) Community psychiatric nurses for the elderly: few side-effects and effective in the treatment of depression. *Journal of Clinical Nursing* **3**:299–306.

Weatherall M. (2000) A randomised controlled trial of the Geriatric Depression Scale in an inpatient ward for older adults. *Clinical Rehabilitation* **14**:186–91.

Whooley MA, Browner WS. (1999) Association between depressive symptoms and mortality in older women. Study of osteoporotic fractures Research Group. *Archives of Internal Medicine* **158**:2129–35.

Whooley MA, Grady D, Cauley JA. (2000) Postmenopausal estrogen therapy and depressive symptoms in older women. *Journal of General Internal Medicine* **15**:535–41.

Wiart L, Petit H, Joseph PA et al. (2000) Fluoxetine in early post-stroke depression: a double-blind placebo-controlled study. *Stroke* **31**:1829–32.

Williams JW, Barrett J, Oxman T et al. (2000) Treatment of dysthymia and minor depression in primary care: a randomised controlled trial in older adults. *Journal of the American Medical Association* **284**:1519–26.

Wilson K, Mottram P, Sivanranthan A, Nightingale A. (2001) Antidepressant versus placebo for depressed elderly (Cochrane Review). In: *The Cochrane Library*, Issue 2, Oxford: Update Software.

Wilson KC, Copeland JR, Taylor S, Donoghue J, McCracken CF. (1999) Natural history of pharmacotherapy of older depressed community residents: the MRC-ALPHA Study. *British Journal of Psychiatry* **175**:439–43.

World Health Organization. (1993) *The ICD-10 Classification of Mental and Behavioural Disorders: Research Criteria*. Geneva, 1993.

Wu LT, Anthony JC. (2000) The estimated rate of depressed mood in US adults: recent evidence for a peak in later life. *Journal of Affective Disorders* **60**:159–71.

Yesavage JA, Brink TL, Rose TL, Lum O. (1983) Development and validation of a geriatric depression screening scale: a preliminary report. *Journal of Psychiatric Research* **17**:37–49.

Yohannes AM, Baldwin RC, Connolly MJ. (2000) Depression and anxiety in elderly outpatients with chronic obstructive pulmonary disease: prevalence and validation of the BASDEC screening questionnaire. *International Journal of Geriatric Psychiatry* **15**:1090–6.

appendix C

Useful textbooks

Baldwin RC. (2002) Depressive disorders. In: Jacoby R, Oppenheimer C, eds. *Psychiatry of Old Age*, 3rd edn. Oxford: Oxford University Press.

Blazer DG. (2002) *Depression in Late Life*, 3rd edn. New York: Springer Verlag.

Curran S, Lynch S, Wattis JP. (2001) *Practical Management of Depression in Older People*. London: Arnold.

Katona CLE. (1994) *Depression in Old Age*. Chichester: John Wiley & Sons.

appendix D

Cognitive Impairment Test

Item	Max Error	Score	Weight
1. What year is it now?	1	_______	× 4 – _______
2. What month is it now?	1	_______	× 3 = _______
Memory Phrase Repeat this phrase after me: Mr John Brown, 42 West Street, Sheffield			
3. What time is it? (Within one hour)	1	_______	× 3 = _______
4. Count backwards 20 to 1	2	_______	× 2 = _______
5. Say the months in reverse order	2	_______	× 2 = _______
6. Repeat the memory phrase	5	_______	× 2 = _______
		Total	= _______

Score of 1 for each incorrect response; maximum weighted error source = 28

Score: 0–11 indicates normal or mild impairment
11–28 indicates moderate to severe impairment

Katzman R, Brown T, Fuld P et al. *American Journal of Psychiatry*, **140**:734–9, 1983.
© 1983, The American Psychiatric Association. http://ajp.psychiatryonline.org
Reprinted by permission.

appendix E

The Hamilton Rating Scale for Depression

1. DEPRESSED MOOD (sadness, hopeless, helpless, worthless)
    - 0 = Absent
    - 1 = These feeling states indicated only on questioning
    - 2 = These feeling states spontaneously reported verbally
    - 3 = Communicates feeling states non-verbally, i.e. through facial expression, posture, voice, and tendency to weep
    - 4 = Patients reports VIRTUALLY ONLY these feeling states in his spontaneous verbal and non-verbal communication

2. FEELINGS OF GUILT
    - 0 = Absent
    - 1 = Self reproach
    - 2 = Ideas of guilt or rumination over past errors or sinful deeds
    - 3 = Present illness is a punishment. Delusions of guilt
    - 4 = Hears accusatory or denunciatory voices and/or experiences threatening visual hallucinations

3. SUICIDE
    - 0 = Absent
    - 1 = Feels life is not worth living
    - 2 = Wishes he were dead or any thoughts of possible death to self
    - 3 = Suicide ideas or gestures
    - 4 = Attempts at suicide (any serious attempts rates 4)

4. INSOMNIA EARLY

0 = No difficulty falling asleep

1 = Complains of occasional difficulty falling asleep – i.e. more than 1½ hour

2 = Complains of nightly difficulty falling asleep

5. INSOMNIA MIDDLE

0 = No difficulty

1 = Patient complains of being restless and disturbed during the night

2 = Waking during the night – any getting out of bed rates 2 (except for the purposed of voiding)

6. INSOMNIA LATE

0 = No difficulty

1 = Waking in early hours of the morning but goes back to sleep

2 = Unable to fall asleep again if he gets out of bed

7. WORK AND ACTIVITIES

0 = No difficulties

1 = Thoughts and feelings of incapacity, fatigue or weakness related to activities; work or hobbies

2 = Loss of interest in activity; hobbies or work – either directly reported by patient, or indirect in listlessness, indecision and vacillation (feels he has to push self to work or activities)

3 = Decrease in actual time spent in activities or decrease in productivity. In hospital rate 3 if patient does not spend at least 3 hours a day in activities (hospital job or hobbies) exclusive of ward chores

4 = Stopped working because of present illness. In hospital, rate 4 if patient engages in no activities except ward chores, or if patient fails to perform ward chores unassisted

8. RETARDATION

0 = Normal speech and thought
1 = Slight retardation at interview
2 = Obvious retardation at interview
3 = Interview difficult
4 = Complete stupor

9. AGITATION

0 = None
1 = Fidgetiness
2 = Playing with hands, hair etc.
3 = Moving about, can't sit still
4 = Hand wringing, nail biting, hair pulling, biting of lips

10. ANXIETY PSYCHIC

0 = No difficulty
1 = Subjective tension and irritability
2 = Worrying about minor matters
3 = Apprehensive attitude apparent in face or speech
4 = Fears expressed without questioning

11. ANXIETY SOMATIC

0 = Absent Psychological concomitants of anxiety such as:
1 = Mild *Gastrointestinal* – dry mouth, wind, indigestion, diarrhoea
2 = Moderate cramps, belching
3 = Severe *Cardiovascular* – palpitations, headaches
4 = Incapacitating *Respiratory* – hyperventilation, sighing, *urinary frequency, sweating*

12. SOMATIC SYMPTOMS GASTROINTESTINAL

0 = None
1 = Loss of appetite but eating without staff encouragement. Heavy feeling in abdomen
2 = Difficulty eating without prompting. Requests or requires laxatives or medication for bowels or medication for gastrointestinal symptoms

13. SOMATIC SYMPTOMS GENERAL

0 = None

1 = Heaviness in limbs, back or head. Backaches, headache, muscle aches. Low energy and fatiguability

2 = Any clear-cut symptoms rates 2

14. GENITAL SYMPTOMS

0 = Absent Symptoms such as: Loss of libido

1 = Mild Menstrual disturbances

2 = Severe

15. HYPOCHONDRIASIS

0 = Not present

1 = Self-absorption (bodily)

2 = Preoccupation with health

3 = Frequent complaints, requests for help etc.

4 = Hypochondriacal delusions

16. LOSS OF WEIGHT Rate either A or B

A. *When rating by history:*

0 = No weight loss

1 = Probably weight loss associated with present illness

2 = Definite (according to patient) weight loss

B. *On weekly ratings, when actual weight changes are measured:*

0 = Less than 0.5 kg weight loss in week

1 = Greater than 0.5 kg weight loss in week

2 = Greater than 1 kg weight loss in week

17. INSIGHT

0 = Acknowledges being depressed and ill

1 = Acknowledges illness but attributes cause to bad food, climate, overwork, virus, need for rest etc.

2 = Denies being ill at all

Note: Moderate depression usually indicated by a score of 18 or greater.

Reproduced from Hamilton M. A rating scale for depression. *Journal of Neurology, Neurosurgery and Psychiatry* (1960) **23**: 56–62, with permission of the BMJ Publishing Group.

appendix F

Montgomery–Asberg Depression Rating Scale

1. Apparent sadness. Reflected in speech, facial expression and posture. Rate by depth and inability to brighten up.

0 No sadness.

1

2 Looks dispirited but does brighten up without difficulty.

3

4 Appears sad and unhappy most of the time.

5

6 Looks miserable all the time. Extremely despondent.

2. Reported sadness. Representing reports of depressed mood, regardless of whether it is reflected in appearance or not. Includes low spirits, despondency or the feeling of being beyond help and without hope. Rate according to intensity, duration and the extent to which the mood is reported to be influenced by events.

0 Occasional sadness in keeping with the circumstances.

1

2 Sad or low but brightens up without difficulty.

3

4 Pervasive feelings of sadness or gloominess. The mood is still influenced by external circumstances.

5

6 Continuous or unvarying sadness, misery or despondency.

3. *Inner tension.* Representing feelings of ill-defined discomfort, edginess, inner turmoil, mental tension mounting to either panic, dread or anguish. Rate according to intensity, frequency, duration and the extent of reassurance called for.

0 Placid. Only fleeting inner tension.
1
2 Occasional feelings of edginess and ill-defined discomfort.
3
4 Continuous feelings of inner tension or intermittent panic which the patient can only master with some difficulty.
5
6 Unrelenting dread or anguish. Overwhelming panic.

4. *Reduced sleep.* Representing the experience of reduced duration or depth of sleep compared to the subject's own normal pattern when well.

0 Sleeps as usual.
1
2 Slight difficulty dropping off to sleep or slightly reduced, light or fitful sleep.
3
4 Sleep reduced or broken by at least 2 hours.
5
6 Less than 2 or 3 hours' sleep.

5. *Reduced appetite.* Representing the feeling of a loss of appetite compared with when well. Rate by loss of desire for food or the need to force oneself to eat.

0 Normal or increased appetite.
1
2 Slightly reduced appetite.
3
4 No appetite. Food is tasteless.
5
6 Needs persuasion to eat at all.

6. Concentration difficulties. Representing difficulties in collecting one's thoughts mounting to incapacitating lack of concentration. Rate according to intensity, frequency, and degree of incapacity produced.

0 No difficulties in concentrating.
1
2 Occasional difficulties in collecting one's thoughts.
3
4 Difficulties in concentrating and sustaining thought which reduces ability to read or hold a conversation.
5
6 Unable to read or converse without great difficulty.

7. Lassitude. Representing a difficulty getting started or slowness initiating and performing everyday activities.

0 Hardly any difficulty in getting started. No sluggishness.
1
2 Difficulties in starting activities.
3
4 Difficulties in starting simple routine activities, which are carried out with effort.
5
6 Complete lassitude. Unable to do anything without help.

8. Inability to feel. Representing the subjective experience of reduced interest in the surroundings, or activities that normally give pleasure. The ability to react with adequate emotion to circumstances or people is reduced.

0 Normal interest in the surroundings and in other people.
1
2 Reduced ability to enjoy usual interests.
3
4 Loss of interest in the surroundings. Loss of feelings for friends and acquaintances.
5
6 The experience of being emotionally paralysed, inability to feel anger, grief or pleasure and a complete or even painful failure to feel for close relatives and friends.

9. Pessimistic thoughts. Representing thoughts of guilt, inferiority, self-reproach, sinfulness, remorse and ruin.

0 No pessimistic thoughts.
1
2 Fluctuating ideas of failure, self-reproach or self-depreciation.
3
4 Persistent self-accusations, or definite but still rational ideas of guilt or sin. Increasingly pessimistic about the future.
5
6 Delusions of ruin, remorse or unredeemable sin. Self-accusations which are absurd and unshakable.

10. Suicidal thoughts. Representing the feeling that life is not worth living, that a natural death would be welcome, suicidal thoughts, and preparations for suicide. Suicidal attempts should not in themselves influence the rating.

0 Enjoys life or takes it as it comes.
1
2 Weary of life. Only fleeting suicidal thoughts.
3
4 Probably better off dead. Suicidal thoughts are common, and suicide is considered as a possible solution, but without specific plans or intention.
5
6 Explicit plans for suicide when there is an opportunity. Active preparations for suicide.

Note: Moderate depression usually indicated by a score of 20 or greater.

Reproduced from the *British Journal of Psychiatry*, **134**, Montgomery SA, Åsberg M, A new depression scale designed to be sensitive to change, 382–9. © 1979 with permission from the Royal College of Psychiatrists

appendix G

Geriatric Depression Scale

Instructions: Choose the best answer for how you have felt over the past *week*.

*1. **Are you basically satisfied with your life?** No
2. **Have you dropped many of your activities and interests?** Yes
*3. **Do you feel your life is empty?** Yes
4. **Do you often get bored?** Yes
5. Are you hopeful about the future? No
6. Are you bothered by thoughts you can't get out of your head? Yes
7. **Are you in good spirits most of the time?** No
*8. **Are you afraid something bad is going to happen to you?** Yes
*9. **Do you feel happy most of the time?** No
10. **Do you often feel helpless?** Yes
11. Do you often get restless and fidgety? Yes
12. **Do you prefer to stay at home, rather than going out and doing new things?** Yes
13. Do you frequently worry about the future? Yes
14. **Do you feel you have more problems with your memory than most?** Yes
15. **Do you think it is wonderful to be alive now?** No

16. Do you often feel down-hearted and blue (sad)? Yes
17. **Do you feel pretty worthless the way you are?** Yes
18. Do you worry a lot about the past? Yes
19. Do you find life very exciting? No
20. Is it hard for you to start on new projects (plans)? Yes
21. **Do you feel full of energy?** No
22. **Do you feel that your situation is hopeless?** Yes
23. **Do you think most people are better off (in their lives) than you are?** Yes
24. Do you frequently get upset over little things? Yes
25. Do you frequently feel like crying? Yes
26. Do you have trouble concentrating? Yes
27. Do you enjoy getting up in the morning? No
28. Do you prefer to avoid social gatherings (get-togethers)? Yes
29. Is it easy for you to make decisions? No
30. Is your mind as clear as it used to be? No

Notes (1) Answers refer to responses which score '1'; (2) bracketed phrases refer to alternative ways of expressing the questions; (3) questions in bold comprise the 15-item version. Cut-off scores for possible depression: >/=11 (GDS30); >/=5 (GDS15); >=2 (GDS4).

* 4-item GDS questions

Reprinted from the *Journal of Psychiatric Research*, **17**, Yesavage JA, Brink TL, Rose TL et al, Development and validation of a geriatric depression screening scale: a preliminary report, 37–49. © 1983 with permission from Elsevier Science.

Index

Note: Page numbers in *italics* refer to boxes in the text